T0098530

BASIC HEALTH PUBLICATIONS USER'S GUIDE

TO GLUCOSAMINE & CHONDROITIN

Don't Be a Dummy. Become an Expert on What Glucosamine & Chondroitin Can Do for Your Health.

VICTORIA DOLBY TOEWS

JACK CHALLEM Series Editor

The information contained in this book is based upon the research and personal and professional experiences of the author. It is not intended as a substitute for consulting with your physician or other health care provider. Any attempt to diagnose and treat an illness should be done under the direction of a health care professional.

The publisher does not advocate the use of any particular health care protocol but believes the information in this book should be available to the public. The publisher and author are not responsible for any adverse effects or consequences resulting from the use of the suggestions, preparations, or procedures discussed in this book. Should the reader have any questions concerning the appropriateness of any procedures or preparation mentioned, the author and the publisher strongly suggest consulting a professional health care advisor.

Series Editor: Jack Challem
Editor: Roberta W. Waddell
Typesetter: Gary A. Rosenberg
Series Cover Designer: Mike Stromberg

Basic Health Publications User's Guides are published by Basic Health Publications, Inc.

Copyright © 2002 by Victoria Dolby Toews

ISBN: 978-1-59120-005-5 (Pbk.)
ISBN: 978-1-68162-855-4 (Hardcover)

CONTENTS

To my husand, Jeff.

With luck (and a handful of supplements)
we'll still be walking the couple of miles,
hand in hand, to the coffee shop
on Sunday mornings
when we are 90.

INTRODUCTION

If you have osteoarthritis, you've got company. Osteoarthritis, the most common form of arthritis, affects about 21 million Americans, giving this disease the dubious distinction of being more common than heart disease or diabetes. And these numbers are on the verge of ballooning as the Baby Boomers are firmly entrenched in the middle-aged years, with the achy joints to prove it. In fact, by the year 2020, the number of those with osteoarthritis is expected to hit 30 million.

The sad truth is that going to your doctor's office is unlikely to result in lasting relief from your joint complaints. In short, conventional medicine has failed many with arthritis. In fact, the side effects of doctor-prescribed medications, such as non-steroidal anti-inflammatory drugs (NSAIDs) that are used to mask the pain of osteoarthritis, often rival the discomfort of the disease itself. To add insult to injury, NSAIDs (the most commonly prescribed drug for osteoarthritis) can, in some cases, even promote additional joint damage. And to date, conventional medicine has nothing to offer in terms of a medication that repairs or rebuilds an osteoarthritic joint.

This is where the natural dietary supplements glucosamine and chondroitin come in. As mentioned, conventional medicine—at best—only addresses the symptoms of osteoarthritis. The crucial difference with glucosamine and chondroitin is that, for the first time, there is a remedy available which actually reverses the damage of osteoarthritis, getting to the source of the problem and repairing joint cartilage.

With glucosamine and chondroitin, you feel better not just because your symptoms are masked, but because your joints are growing new and healthy cartilage to cushion the space where bones meet. While neither promise to be magic bullets, more often than not they succeed in reducing the pain and impairment of mobility in arthritis.

Perhaps you've been intrigued by natural remedies' claims for aiding health woes such as osteoarthritis, but worry that it's "too good to be true." Think again. Scientifically based clinical trials are stacking up in favor of the ability of glucosamine and chondroitin to provide real relief for aching joints.

It can be hard to get the real scoop about dietary supplements. Some things you read are just hype, overstating the value of a particular supplement with the goal to simply sell more bottles, while other sources are overly skeptical of any supplements and dismiss them all as a waste of money. It's time that the plain truth is told.

This *User's Guide to Glucosamine & Chondroitin* provides straightforward information—not hype—about glucosamine and chondroitin. Chapter 1 starts with the basics of understanding the problem of osteoarthritis and how your joints are damaged by this condition. Chapter 2 puts this into perspective by explaining how glucosamine and chondroitin can provide symptom relief and rebuild damaged cartilage. Realistic information about how you can expect to feel while taking these joint-friendly supplements is found here, too.

Subsequent chapters share the history and development of glucosamine and chondroitin, as well as the nuts and bolts of how to use glucosamine and chondroitin dietary supplements and information about a handful of additional supplements that aid in joint recovery. The role of conventional medications, such as NSAIDs will also be explored. Other health conditions, such as heart disease and migraines, can benefit from glucosamine and chondroitin; these will be discussed in Chapter 7. Finally, the book will touch on minor safety concerns with the use of these supplements to ensure that you get the maximum benefit, with the minimum risk, from choosing these dietary supplements.

Isn't it time that you found relief for your osteoarthritis? Read on to finally find an osteoarthritis remedy that offers a long-term solution to your ailment.

CHAPTER 1

JOINTS IN TROUBLE

Osteoarthritis is no fun at all. It's a thief that can take away your ability to be fully engaged in daily activities. As it progresses, you might have days you can't even get out of bed. It is one of the oldest and most common diseases suffered by humans. Arthritis can hit only one joint, which is especially common in the early stages of the disease, or it may affect many joints in the body. In addition, arthritis can vary in severity from a mild ache and stiffness to crippling pain and even joint deformity.

What, Exactly, Is Osteoarthritis?

Osteoarthritis is a medical disease name created from Greek terms, with "osteo" referring to bones, "arthro" indicating that joints are involved, and "itis" meaning inflammation. This is actually somewhat of a misnomer, since pain is the hallmark feature of this condition while inflammation is only rarely implicated, although it certainly involves the bones and joints. Osteoarthritis is a chronic disease involving the breakdown of the joints and surrounding tissues.

In osteoarthritis, the problem lies with the cartilage that protects the ends of bones. This cartilage is a necessary cushion between bones and when it wears away, the bones grinding together cause the common complaints of stiffness and pain. As such, osteoarthritis is the leading cause of disability.

Quality of Life
Osteoarthritis can have a huge impact on the quality of life. About 100,000 people in the United States alone are estimated to be unable to walk because of severe osteoarthritis in the hip or knee.

Osteoarthritis comes in two "flavors." Primary osteoarthritis is the more prevalent flavor, and it is a slow, but progressive, type of osteoarthritis that generally develops after age forty-five. With primary osteoarthritis, the knees and hips are the main target. The exact cause of primary osteoarthritis is not known, although obesity and family history of this disease do play a role.

Secondary osteoarthritis, on the other hand, can be traced to a specific cause. In many cases, this cause was a traumatic event, such as a sports injury, that left the joint vulnerable. In other cases, it can be related to joint infection, surgery of the joint, or chronic trauma. An example of chronic trauma would be a repetitive motion that damages the joint, such as a baseball pitcher repeatedly throwing a ball. Most younger people with osteoarthritis have secondary osteoarthritis.

How Joints Work

Joints, as the name implies, are the point at which two bones meet. And the human body has over 100 different joints. The joints of the body are known as the articulation system and are responsible for the body's ability to move.

There are three kinds of joints in the body, each with different movement capabilities. The three joint types are cartilaginous, fibrous, and synovial. The synovial joints, including elbows, fingers, hips, and knees, are the most complex since they allow for the greatest movement. The cartilaginous joints, such as the joints between ribs, are slightly movable. The fibrous joints, such as the bones of the skull, are generally immovable.

Osteoarthritis overwhelmingly favors the highly movable synovial joints (although cartilaginous joints very occasionally develop osteoarthritis). The term synovial joint reflects the fact that these joints contain synovial fluid. This clear, sticky fluid lubricates the joints for ease of movement and is produced in the synovial membrane which lines the joint. Synovial fluid is very important for healthy joints because cartilage does not have its own blood supply. This fluid supplies the building blocks for the repair of cartilage and removes waste products.

Synovial Joints Are Ground Zero

Synovial joints, such as those of the knee and hip, are highly movable joints and are the joints most frequently affected by osteoarthritis.

Cartilage Is the Key to Healthy Joints

Cartilage acts as a smooth, slippery surface so the bones can move easily past one another. It's the layer of resilient tissue cushioning the ends of bones where joints meet that allows flexible movement and absorbs shock. Cartilage is made up of three primary substances: collagen (a special kind of protein), proteoglycans (compounds made of protein and sugar), and water. You may already be familiar with collagen, since it is also the building block of bone, skin, tendon, and other connective tissues.

A mesh network of collagen fibers forms the framework of cartilage. Proteoglycans work and act like miniature sponges to trap water within the cartilage structure. This trapped water is what allows cartilage to absorb shock and spring back after being compressed during the normal movements of a joint.

What is cartilage?

Cartilage is mostly water. It also contains a special type of protein called collagen that forms a mesh framework. Attached to this framework are protein-sugar compounds that trap the water to give cartilage its resiliency.

Additionally, cartilage also contains cells called chondrocytes, which manufacture new collagen and proteoglycans, as well as secrete enzymes to degrade old collagen and proteoglycan molecules. In other words, chondrocytes are the birthplace of both the collagen and proteoglycans that, in turn, create cartilage. Sometimes these chondrocytes malfunction and the balance between the degrading enzymes and the rebuilding process is disturbed. In addition, the new proteoglycans that are made in the malfunctioning chondrocytes are sometimes incomplete and defective, which means they are simply not up to the important job of contributing to strong, resilient cartilage. When these things happen, the stage can be set for osteoarthritis.

The spongelike qualities of cartilage are due in large part to the fact that cartilage contains up to 80 percent water. This unique blend of collagen, proteoglycans, and water means that joints of the body are able to absorb the shock of walking, running, jumping, and all other manner of activities. In fact, for someone who weighs 200 pounds, the weight-bearing joints (knees and hips) have to sustain up to a ton of pressure during active use. Ideally, the joints can handle this load, but joints with osteoarthritis are simply not up to the challenge and regular activities can become painful.

> **The Many Faces of Cartilage**
>
> *Cartilage is a pretty amazing substance. It is hard, yet elastic in its response to mechanical stress. It is also able to absorb tremendous shock but has a surface smoothness that exceeds the slipperiness of ice.*

The Osteoarthritic Joint

You've just read how the inside of a healthy joint looks. Now let's take a look inside a joint with osteoarthritis. In the early stages, the first thing that happens is an increase in the enzymes that break down proteoglycans. Unfortunately, the creation of new proteoglycans just can't keep pace with the destruction and, without them, collagen fibers become exposed. Not normally exposed, these fibers are now attacked by enzymes, degrading them further.

In the final stages of arthritis developing in the joint, the entire cartilage matrix has been dissolved, the chondrocytes are disappearing, and the ends of bones are exposed and rubbing painfully together. In addition, the area becomes inflamed as the body tries to protect the joint. However, this inflammation contributes to the breakdown of tissue and this, in turn, promotes more pain in the joint.

Who Gets Osteoarthritis?

With age comes wisdom, and also—for many of us—osteo- arthritis. This joint disease gener- ally sets in after age forty and is the most common source of physical disability in adults. With increasing age, the risk of osteo - arthritis rises dramatically. On av- erage, each year after age forty, there's a 2 percent rise in the rate of osteoarthritis. Looking at the population as a whole, 21 million Americans can be counted among those with osteoarthritis.

Joints at Risk for Osteoarthritis
Osteoarthritis could theoretically strike any of the body's joints, but it most often affects the feet, fingers, hips, knees, lower back, and neck, rarely the elbows or shoulders.

By age sixty-five, the average person getting an x-ray of a weight-bearing joint would have a 50 per- cent chance of learning they have osteoarthritis. Since the numbers of Americans reaching age fifty- five and beyond is increasing, so too are the num- bers of people developing osteoarthritis.

Lots of people younger than forty develop this joint condition as well, but their cases can generally be traced to a specific joint injury. Both men and women have this disease. Before age forty-five, however, more men have it, while after age forty-five, osteoarthritis is far more common in women.

If you have a close family member with osteoarthritis, your chances of also getting the disease yourself are higher. In addition, being overweight places an extra load on your joints and increases your risk. The connection between obesity and osteoarthritis seems straightforward at first glance, since extra weight makes the weight-bearing joints of the knee and hip work harder. While this is true, it is not yet understood why being overweight also increases the risk of osteoarthritis in the hand. The good news is that weight loss can keep you from getting this disease if you don't yet have it, and if you already do, losing weight helps lessen symptoms.

Secondary osteoarthritis, as previously mentioned, is related to a specific cause. This can include a sports or other injury to a joint, an infection in a joint, a metabolic imbalance (such as calcium deposits), or chronic overuse of a joint from hard labor or sports. In other words, specific stresses on a joint stemming from overuse, trauma, and certain occupations that demand high use from joints, can accelerate the aging of cartilage. It is important to point out here that regular exercise does not cause osteoarthritis and, in fact, does the opposite, since being physically active can help those with osteoarthritis. But it is very important, when working a physical job or when involved in athletics, to be careful that the joints are not overburdened and put at risk for developing secondary osteoarthritis.

What Are the Symptoms?

Osteoarthritis can sneak up on you. It probably started out with one joint (most likely your knee or hip) feeling just a bit stiff in the morning. In general, the pain is asymmetrical, with only the knee or hip on one side of the body being bothered. Over time, however, this can change, with multiple joints developing problems.

What began as morning stiffness can then extend throughout the day in the form of pain, with the affected joint manifesting pain anytime it is used, especially if used actively. The joint will generally feel better with rest. Late in the disease process, however, the joint can be painful with the slightest movement, or even when at rest. Also, as the disease progresses, morning stiffness can occur anytime a joint is not used for a while (such as on a car trip), and the range of motion of the joint can be diminished.

Joint cracking, with both an audible sound and a sensation of crunching, also occurs in the joint. While this can be loud, it is not usually a painful experience.

> **How do I know if it's osteoarthritis?**
> *Pain and morning stiffness of a joint, such as the knee or hip, are the most common signs of osteoarthritis. Limited range of motion is also common.*

Shooting pain down the arms or up the back of the head and down the back of the thighs may result from osteoarthritis and is called *referred pain*. Other possible symptoms are muscle spasms and bony growths (called *nodes*) in the fingers.

Inflammation occasionally occurs with osteoarthritis, but is not the primary symptom. If there is inflammation related to osteoarthritis, it is probably very late in the course of the disease. Inflammation is the hallmark of rheumatoid arthritis, a different form of the disease that is not the focus of this book.

Osteoarthritis is a progressive disease. This means your symptoms will tend to worsen over time. In advanced cases, bone spurs can form and bones can even become deformed.

Just Part of the Aging Process?

Some people assume that osteoarthritis is simply an inevitable part of the aging process due to wear and tear on the joint. In fact, this is why osteoarthritis used to be known as "wear and tear" arthritis. But modern understanding of this condition now shows that osteoarthritis is not just the result of joints worn out by decades of use, but instead is caused when the body's process of maintaining healthy cartilage is no longer functioning properly.

There are a few theories about what goes wrong in the cartilage repair process that leads to osteoarthritis, and several of these may be happening at the same time. In some cases, the chondrocytes that make new cartilage seem to put out the wrong mixture of cartilage ingredients. In other cases, the chondrocytes are sending out too many of the cartilage-destroying enzymes and not enough of the materials needed to build new cartilage.

Key Signs of Osteoarthritis
1. Joint pain, either steady or intermittent.
2. Stiffness in the joint upon first getting out of bed.
3. Joint cracking.
4. Limited range of motion.

It used to be assumed that this malfunctioning of chondrocytes was not reversible. Today, we know this is not necessarily true. Glucosamine and chondroitin provide the help your body needs to correct the process of creating new, healthy cartilage. You'll learn more details about this amazing breakthrough in Chapter 2.

Preventing Arthritis

Arthritis is not inevitable, there are ways to minimize the risk that it will develop, or at least stave off the inevitable for as long as possible. As the saying goes, an ounce of prevention is worth a pound of cure.

The most important tool for preventing most types of arthritis is exercise. The reason for this lies in the unique anatomy of the joint. Joints do not have a blood supply to nourish them, as other body tissues do. Rather, joints get oxygen and nourishment and eliminate waste as the result of joint movement. During motion, synovial fluid is squeezed into the space between joints and then squeezed out. "Use it or lose it" does seem to apply in this situation. Without joint activity and motion, joints become starved for oxygen and other nutrients which contributes to joint degeneration and arthritis.

Exercise, including stretching, strengthening, and aerobics, is a common recommendation for patients with arthritis, but the pain and mobility impairments associated with arthritis often make it difficult for an individual to comply with this advice. Still, it is important to find an exercise, even if it is only slow walking, that is comfortable for your body.

Exercise has several benefits. The bones respond to exercise by growing stronger and becoming better support structures. And improved muscle tone resulting from improved fitness assists in supporting and stabilizing the joints. Keeping active also maintains the health of cartilage, while inactivity leads to cartilage degeneration. Finally, the beneficial psychological effects of exercise help to prevent anxiety and depression. Biking, swimming, and walking are great exercises to start with, but it is very important to begin any exercise program slowly.

Avoiding injuries is another key factor in an arthritis prevention plan. Of course, the nature of injuries is that they are unplanned; nonetheless, there are ways to minimize the risk. For example, wear shoes that fit properly. Shoes that are too tight can damage the toe joints and lead to arthritis. Likewise, certain occupations can lead to joint problems. If the chair of someone who sits all day is not supportive, or if their posture is incorrect, extensive vertebral damage can develop.

The last piece of advice for reducing the risk of arthritis is already well-known to most people: maintain a healthy weight. The strain of extra weight on the weight-bearing joints (hips, knees, and ankles) can actually destroy the joint. Overweight men and women are 30 percent more likely than their normal weight counterparts to have arthritis. The situation gets worse as the pounds add up. Obese men are at 70 percent higher risk and obese women are at 50 percent higher risk of developing arthritis. But the good news is that losing the weight reduces the risk of arthritis.

Diagnosing Arthritis

Finding out whether the ache you feel in your knee, or the catch in your hip is osteoarthritis is not as easy as you would think. There's no single, clear-cut test for osteoarthritis. Instead, your doctor will use a combination of the methods described in this section, as well as ruling out other conditions.

Your doctor will probably start by asking you to describe your symptoms, when they first developed, and how they have changed over time. This is known as a clinical history. Specifically, the doctor will want you to describe any pain, stiffness, and range-of-motion limitation in the affected joint. Next up is a physical examination of the joint to check how impeded the joint usage is.

Osteoarthritis vs. Rheumatoid Arthritis
Osteoarthritis can mimic other health problems. The joint pain and stiffness of rheumatoid arthritis can be very similar, but it is an autoimmune disorder and has a different treatment.

In addition, x-rays may be taken to determine the extent of joint damage. X-rays can show if there has been any cartilage loss, bone damage, or if bone spurs are present. Disease severity as it appears in x-rays does not always closely match how much pain or disability a person with osteoarthritis experiences. Furthermore, early stages of osteoarthritis do not always appear in x-rays.

In order to confirm a diagnosis of arthritis, a physician may use a syringe to extract some fluid from the affected joint and examine it microscopically for the presence of microorganisms, uric acid, or other substances. This fluid may also be cultured in order to analyze it for infections.

Other joint disorders will be ruled out. For instance, blood tests are utilized in some cases to determine the presence of proteins typical of rheumatoid arthritis or high levels of uric acid indicative of gout. Bursitis symptoms can mimic osteoarthritis symptoms, but the treatment would be different.

Once you know you have osteoarthritis, the next natural step is trying to determine how you can regain as much of your health and quality of life as possible. This is where glucosamine and chondroitin enter the picture. The following chapters will focus on how you can use these dietary supplements to reduce your symptoms, and rebuild healthy cartilage in your ailing joints at the same time.

CHAPTER 2

THE CARTILAGE HEALING SOLUTION

Successful treatment of osteoarthritis has two main goals. The first is to control pain, and the second is to slow down—and ideally reverse—the progression of this disease. Conventional medicine has worked hard on this problem, but to date it has only been able to address the first part of this solution—minimizing some of the discomfort that defines osteoarthritis.

Glucosamine and chondroitin are the first well-researched compounds that are meeting both arthritis treatment goals: to control pain *and* to afford some recovery of cartilage function. These supplements don't just ease joint pain and tenderness and improve range of motion, they also promote healing of cartilage.

What Is Glucosamine?

Glucosamine is the fundamental building block for the key cartilage ingredient called proteoglycans. You may recall from the last chapter that proteoglycans act as sponges to contain the water necessary for resilient joints. As the name implies, glucose (sugar) and an amino acid (protein building block) are combined to create "glucosamine." Although the body creates its own glucosamine, in cases of osteoarthritis an extra boost in supply can make a big difference to joint health.

This is one little compound that certainly gets

The Name Game

Glucosamine and chondroitin have been a hot topic of discussion lately, but what's the right way to pronounce these mouthfuls? Glucosamine is pronounced "glue-KOSE-a-meen" and chondroitin is said "kon-DROY-tin."

around. In addition to helping make cartilage in joints, glucosamine is also needed, either directly or indirectly, for the formation of blood vessels, bone, heart valves, ligaments, nails, skin, synovial fluid, tendons, and mucus secretions of the digestive tract. Glucos - amine is also needed by the body to make chondroitin.

Glucosamine taken orally in a capsule is quickly and almost completely (90 percent) absorbed from the GI tract. In processing this compound, the body sends the lion's share to areas of cartilage where it can be used to build new, healthy cartilage in joints.

What Is Chondroitin?

Much like glucosamine, chondroitin is also made within the body and is a necessary component of cartilage and other connective tissues. Chondroitin sulfate, its technical name, belongs to a class of compounds called glycosaminoglycans. Although chondroitin sulfate is often referred to as if it were one thing, there are actually several unique, yet structurally similar, types of this compound. The most abundant in the body are chondroitin-4-sulfate and chondroitin-6-sulfate. The number in each of the names refers to the location of the sulfate molecule along the chondroitin chain.

Because there are slightly different structures of chondroitin sulfate molecules, each of the individual structures has different weights. There has been some discussion amongst chondroitin researchers about how the different weights influence the absorption and use of these compounds. Some evidence indicates that the lower weight compounds are more readily absorbed, but the ideal structure of chondroitin remains unknown.

Unlike glucosamine, chon - droitin is not well absorbed when ingested orally. In fact, the absorption numbers are mirror images of each other: while 90 percent of glucosamine is absorbed, less than 10 percent of chondroitin is absorbed. This absorption issue is still being researched, since there are many factors—such

The Chondroitin Family

Supplements of chondroitin sulfate are actually a group of compounds with very similar structures. The differences involve where the sulfate joins onto the chondroitin molecule which affects how well the body uses each type of chondroitin.

as molecular weight and location of sulfate groups—that affect the absorption of chondroitin. Some experts theorize that low-molecular-mass chondroitin would be better absorbed. There are currently several products on the market that are designed as low molecular mass.

Even without the specific details of what happens to chondroitin molecules after they are swallowed in a supplement, numerous scientific studies have shown that taking chondroitin sulfate as a dietary supplement results in better joint health.

Joint Benefits of Glucosamine

Osteoarthritis causes cartilage to be worn away, but the good news is that glucosamine can help your body rebuild this cartilage. Here's how: when glucosamine is taken as a supplement, most of it ends up in joint tissues. Once in the cartilage, glucosamine enters the chondrocytes, the cartilage-building factories located within the cartilage tissue, and they utilize the glucosamine to create new proteoglycans.

This revved-up manufacture of proteoglycans helps, in turn, to restore healthy joint function. Remember, it is the proteoglycans that trap water and give joints their springy quality. Increased proteoglycan production is important since one of the hallmarks of osteoarthritis is the body's inability to create enough new proteoglycans to keep up with the loss of this cartilage component.

But that's not all. In any body tissue, new cells are constantly being manufactured to take the place of old cells, a cell-replacement process that is facilitated by enzymes that degrade the old cells. Sometimes, however, the enzymatic breakdown of proteoglycans in cartilage occurs more quickly than their replacement by new cells, which can result in fragile and inelastic cartilage. Here's where glucosamine comes in. It inhibits this misguided, too-rapid enzymatic destruction of proteoglycans, in addition to having an anti-inflammatory effect on the joint.

Joint Benefits of Chondroitin

The beneficial role of chondroitin is both similar and complementary to that of glucosamine. For starters, chondroitin also plays an important role in creating new crops of healthy water-trapping proteoglycans. Since it has a negative charge, each of its molecules is slightly pushed apart from nearby molecules to create small spaces within the cartilage matrix which are then filled with water. Both glucosamine and chondroitin have been observed in the laboratory to stimulate the creation of proteoglycans by chondrocytes.

The absorption of water into the cartilage matrix is important, since cartilage has no blood supply of its own and depends on the movement of fluid into cartilage to bring necessary nutrients into the joint. The water that fills the spaces within the proteoglycans also acts as a shock absorber for the compression caused during joint movement.

As previously explained, there are enzymes released within the joint that destroy proteoglycans, preparing the way for new proteoglycans to take their place. In osteoarthritic joints, these enzymes are out of balance with the creation of new proteoglycans.

Getting Enzymes Back in Balance

When too many cartilage-eating enzymes are breaking down joint tissues, chondroitin can help. Chondroitin inhibits these destructive enzymes, while boosting the synthesis of new cartilage tissue.

Chondroitin inhibits several of these degrading enzymes, thereby slowing the out-of-balance destruction of proteoglycans and collagen in cartilage. Italian researchers have documented this in a study which found that the oral use of chondroitin sulfate for five days by one group of individuals with cartilage degeneration and a second group with healthy cartilage significantly decreased the levels of cartilage-degrading enzymes in both groups.

As with glucosamine, chondroitin also has the ability to lessen joint inflammation. Although this is not the core problem in the early stages of osteoarthritis, it can become quite debilitating as the disease progresses. This anti-inflammatory effect of chondroitin (as well as glucosamine) is special because, in contrast to prescribed NSAIDs, it does not alter hormonelike substances in the body called prostaglandins, and their function is allowed to continue unharmed. (In Chapter 6, you'll learn in more detail about how NSAIDs alter prostaglandins in order to quell inflammation, and how this, in turn, can lead to a bevy of side effects, such as stomach upset.)

Helping Cartilage Rebuild Itself

Both glucosamine and chondroitin bring the joint remodeling process back into balance by quelling

Understanding Chondroprotection

"Chondroprotection" is the ability of certain substances to protect the integrity of cartilage. Glucosamine and chondroitin have this chondroprotective ability since they stimulate the metabolism of chondrocytes, the cells which produce collagen and proteoglycans, inhibit the production of enzymes that degrade cartilage, and lessen swelling.

the destructive enzymes and beefing up the proteoglycan-building ability of chondrocytes. What this means, specifically, is that osteoarthritis progression can be stopped in its tracks. A landmark study that brought together arthritis experts from four countries and 212 people with osteoarthritis found irrefutable proof that glucosamine does in fact prevent this disease from progressing.

This study, reported in the prestigious medical journal *Lancet*, adhered to the strictest scientific principles. It was double blind, which means that neither the patients nor the doctors had any idea which person was taking glucosamine and which was taking a placebo (dummy pill). Comparing the glucosamine supplements to a placebo was an important aspect of this study, since it takes away the possibility that any benefit found in this study only occurred because of wishful thinking.

All the patients had osteoarthritis of the knee.

"Double Blind" Means Strong Science

When researchers design a double-blind study, neither the investigator nor the patients know whether they are getting the active treatment or a sham. This means that preconceived ideas about how a treatment might work won't affect the objective results of the study.

Half the people took 1,500 mg of glucosamine sulfate per day, the other half were given a placebo. This supplement regimen was continued for three years, and during that time, pain symptoms increased by 10 percent in the placebo group, but dropped by 20 to 25 percent for the glucosamine sulfate group. Similarly, the placebo group continued to experience worsening knee-joint abnormalities while the glucosamine sulfate group showed no deterioration based on x-ray examinations. This is considered landmark research since it was the first time that glucosamine was documented to stop the progression of this disease.

Another group of researchers, however, were not necessarily surprised by these exciting results, since they had already viewed cartilage that was able to rebuild itself with the help of glucosamine. When scanned electron micrographs of cartilage were examined in their study, people who had taken glucosamine showed evidence that their cartilage was actually rebuilding itself.

Chondroitin supplements share a similar success story. When 226 adults with thinning cartilage were administered oral doses of chondroitin sulfate or an inactive placebo daily for one year, the cartilage of those taking the chondroitin sulfate stopped thinning or even improved in thickness. In addition, the chondroitin sulfate group showed significant improvements in all measured parameters, including pain and joint mobility.

In an exhaustive review and reanalysis of all research related to knee and hip osteoarthritis from 1966 to 1999, researchers publishing in the *Journal of the American Medical Association* concluded that glucosamine and chondroitin do, in fact, show a "moderate to large" effect for easing osteoarthritis symptoms. Coming from such a prestigious publication, it is reassuring news that these supplements are no flash in the pan, but a serious treatment consideration for osteoarthritis.

Good Things Are Worth Waiting For

Researchers conducting studies with glucosamine and chondroitin for osteoarthritis can sometimes sound like broken records because they repeat the same recommendation over and over: glucosamine and chondroitin should be considered as the first-choice, basic therapy for the management of osteoarthritis.

In other words, highly trained researchers recommend that glucosamine/chondroitin should be tried as an osteoarthritis treatment before aspirin, NSAIDs, or surgery. This does not mean that these supplements will completely resolve the disease in every person, but rather that it is the most sensible place to start since the potential for benefit is high and the risk of side effects is exceedingly low.

So how are you likely to feel different after using one or both of these supplements? For starters, you'll need to be prepared to not feel anything for several weeks. Numerous studies have noted the fact that, similar to vitamin and mineral intake, there is a lag time before glucosamine and chondroitin cause changes that can be felt. For instance, most people with osteoarthritis who take ibuprofen, the NSAID pain reliever, notice some pain relief within a week of use, whereas it might take several weeks before glucosamine/chondroitin approaches the pain relief afforded by an NSAID.

Experts Agree: Try Glucosamine and Chondroitin First

Osteoarthritis experts repeatedly state in research articles that these supple - ments should be the first treatment attempted for osteoarthritis.

Hang in there, though, because in just a couple more weeks of use, the glucosamine/chondroitin users will usually have surpassed the pain relief of the ibuprofen users. Although it will likely take at least one solid month of daily use before glucosamine and chondroitin will exert their full benefit, it's a classic case of "good things being worth waiting for." This time lag is understandable once you realize that glucosamine/chondroitin are not just applying Band-Aids, they are working to root out the cause of the problem by rebuilding the joint structure, and it takes time to create new, healthy tissue.

While an escape from pain and discomfort is very welcome indeed, it is not the only change the typical user of glucosamine and/or chondroitin experiences. Taking these supplements helps to reduce the swelling of an inflamed joint and lessens the nagging sensation of stiffness in the joints, primarily in the morning, but also any time a joint hasn't been used in a while. People who take glucosamine/chondroitin report being able to more fully move their affected joint through its normal range, while others report an improved walking speed as one more benefit of these supplements.

So that's what to expect if you take them. But what if you choose not to? The science on this is clear. Untreated osteoarthritis is a progressively worsening condition, and you will most likely feel worse as time goes by.

For example, in one study comparing glucosamine to a placebo (dummy pill), those taking glucosamine had a 24 percent decrease in their symptom scores, but the placebo group's symptom score *increased* by 10 percent. Furthermore, according to x-rays of their knees, the glucosamine group showed no further joint deterioration, but the placebo group continued to show a significant increase in abnormalities. There is definitely a risk involved if you choose to do nothing about your osteoarthritis.

Getting to the Source of the Problem

Treatments for osteoarthritis are generally divided into two categories: symptom-modifying and structure-modifying. As yet, no prescription or over-the-counter medication has been found to be in the latter category. All that doctors have in their current arsenal to mask some of the symptoms of osteoarthritis are drugs, namely NSAIDs. But that's not all. Some of the NSAIDs in common use by conventional medicine are actually known to *worsen* the progression of osteoarthritis.

Fortunately there is glucosamine and chondroitin. These supplements qualify as both symptom-modifying and structure-modifying. Not only do these natural remedies mask osteoarthritis symptoms, they are actually the only remedy yet found to favorably modify the structure of the joint. In short, it's the answer that millions of people with osteoarthritis have been waiting for: a remedy to ease discomfort and heal the joint.

Here are five key ways that glucosamine and chondroitin act as both symptom-modifying and structure-modifying agents for osteoarthritis treatment. They:

1. Reduce joint pain and swelling.

2. Increase water content of cartilage.

3. Slow down action of cartilage-eating enzymes.

4. Step up production of new cartilage components (proteoglycans and collagen).

5. Improve viscosity of synovial fluid (joint lubrication).

Putting Glucosamine/Chondroitin to the Test

The National Center for Complementary and Alternative Medicine and the National Institute of Arthritis and Musculoskeletal Disease are funding a $14-million study to examine whether glucosamine and chondroitin supplements can ease the pain of osteoarthritis.

This study—the Glucosamine/Chondroitin Arthritis Intervention Trial (GAIT)—will last for twenty-four weeks and enroll almost 1,600 patients at thirteen different clinical centers. The efficacy of glucosamine and chondroitin alone, in combination, compared to a placebo, and compared to a conventional medication (celecoxib) for relieving osteoarthritic knee pain will be measured.

The trial will continue with a subset of the participants for another eighteen months to assess how the supplements might alter the progression of the osteoarthritis. The final results of this ambitious study won't be available until 2005. You probably won't want to wait until then, however, to give these great supplements a try.

CHAPTER 3

A Star
Is Born

The United States is generally thought of as a leader in science and medicine, but in the case of alternative medicine, we are playing catch-up. Many other countries are researching and using natural therapies at a much higher rate than the U.S., and glucosamine and chondroitin are a case in point.

Glucosamine Enters the Scene

You may be hearing about glucosamine for the first time, but it is by no means a "new" supplement. Glucosamine is a substance naturally made by and found in the human body. The synthesis of glucos-amine sulfate was first described by a chemist back in 1898. However, it took until relatively recently to develop a more stable compound with a long shelf life. Today, supplements of glucosamine are made from chitin, a source material found in crab, shrimp, and lobster shells.

**Glucosamine
Could Be Considered
a Nutrient**
Glucosamine is made by the body, and is naturally found in meat, poultry, and fish. The body readily absorbs and uses the small amounts of glucosamine from food sources, and for this reason some experts suggest that it could legitimately be considered a nutrient.

Scientists first got an inkling that glucosamine could play a role in joint problems about half a century ago. Laboratory studies using petri dishes of cartilage cells found that the addition of glucosamine kicked the secretion of glycosaminoglycans and collagen into high gear. A few years later, in 1969, glucosamine was documented to relieve human patients with osteoarthritis. German researchers used an injectable form of glucosamine sulfate to bring about reductions in pain and improve mobility. These first human studies, however, were not controlled, meaning that no placebo was used and the study was not double blind, so there was always a chance that the promising results were actually a result of wishful thinking on the part of the patients or doctors.

Over the next two decades, several controlled studies were published by researchers from several countries (including Italy, Portugal, and the Philippines) which showed that glucosamine really does aid joint health. During this time, the U.S. virtually ignored the building body of research in favor of glucosamine, even though the results of these studies uniformly found that glucosamine reduced joint pain and improved range of motion in affected joints.

Veterinarians Use These Supplements, Too
Glucosamine and chondroitin are increasingly used in veterinary medicine to treat arthritis in dogs, horses, and other animals. In fact, this has been a common practice in Europe for several decades.

In time, an Italian pharmaceutical company developed glucosamine in an oral (pill) form much preferred by patients to the injected form. The standard dose was established as 1,500 mg. The body of research documenting the benefits of glucosamine continued to grow, and the low incidence of side effects from this supplement became irrefutable.

Chondroitin Makes Its Mark

Chondroitin was first identified as a component of

cartilage in the 1940s. Supplements of chondroitin sulfate use cartilage from pigs, chicken, fish, and cows as a source material. Regarding the latter, there have been concerns raised about the risk of mad cow disease (bovine spongiform encephalopathy) contaminating chondroitin supplements. Chapter 8 discusses this concern in more detail, but the bottom line is that supplement manufacturers take the same steps as companies producing beef products to ensure that this animal-based product has an extremely low risk for transmitting this disease.

The early research with chondroitin primarily used this supplement in animals to demonstrate its application for joint health. Other laboratory research on animals showed that chondroitin increases proteoglycan production. Trials involving people with osteoarthritis soon followed and, as with glucosamine, this supplement was repeatedly shown to relieve joint pain, improve mobility, lessen swelling, increase walk time, and decrease the use of NSAID medications.

The Overlooked Medical Miracle

Although glucosamine is a mainstay treatment for osteoarthritis in Europe, and has been for years, glucosamine and chondroitin have only recently become commonplace in the United States. What accounts for this disparity in how osteoarthritis is treated on either side of the Atlantic? To find the answer to this question, one simply needs to "follow the money."

Pharmaceutical companies spend an enormous amount of money researching and marketing drugs to treat diseases. The way they recoup all this outflow of money is by investing in drugs they can patent. Patented medicines, such as the NSAID medications, are protected and allow the patent holder to corner the market and charge higher prices than are charged for a product produced by competitive manufacturers.

While this situation leads to the development of some very useful and life-saving medications, it does have the downfall that products like nutrition-al supplements which can-not be patented are often left by the wayside. Thus, the medical-pharmaceuti-cal industry ignores these natural agents because there is no money to be made. Instead they turn out, one after another, new drugs, such as Cox-2 in-hibitors that drain pocket-books, and rack up unfor-tunate side effects.

Patents Shape Our "Medicine Chests"

Glucosamine and chondroitin are natural products that cannot be patented. This means that medical companies lack the financial-payoff incentive to pour money into research and promotion campaigns. Thus, you may only be hearing about these valuable treatments for osteoarthritis for the first time in this book.

There simply isn't as ready a source of research dollars to study nutritional supplements as there is for pharmaceuticals. This doesn't mean that nutri-tional supplements lack amazing potential for heal-ing, it just means they lack funding.

But this has been changing. Overall, there is growing interest in natural healing modalities. With the rise of the Internet, more of the international re-search on glucosamine and chondroitin has gotten attention, and more physicians are becoming open to the use of dietary supplements.

For glucosamine and chondroitin, the biggest moment of change came in 1997 when a book called *The Arthritis Cure* took the morning news programs, newspapers, and the awareness of the general public by storm. The authors of this book, Dr. Jason Theodosakis, Brenda Adderly, and Dr. Barry Fox, contended that glucosamine and chon-droitin could halt, reverse, and even cure osteo -

arthritis. It truly caused a groundswell of interest in these supplements by the average person that could no longer be ignored. Overnight, glucosamine became a household word. Since then, much more has been learned about using these supplements.

Quality Control Remains Strong

You shell out the money for a bottle of pills, but how do you really know what's in those pills? In the case of glucosamine and chondroitin, you don't have to worry. Although there has been in-fighting between supplement companies accusing each other of putting out poor-quality products, the bottom line seems to be that the average bottle of glucosamine/chondroitin really is of high quality.

A non-profit organization related to the natural products industry put twenty-eight brands of glucosamine to the test. All the supplement bottles were randomly purchased from stores, and then sent to independent laboratories for analysis of the amount and type of glucosamine. To achieve a passing score, the products needed to pass both tests within a 5 percent margin of error. Every single product passed, which indicated that it contained exactly what the label listed in terms of product type and quantity.

Glucosamine Passes Independent Quality Control Testing
All twenty-eight bottles of glucosamine tested by an independent laboratory were found to contain the amount of glucosamine advertised on the label, and the type of glucosamine listed in the ingredients.

This should give glucosamine users peace of mind that they are getting what they paid for.

Costs of Supplementation

Consumers spend about $400 million on glucosamine and chondroitin supplements annually. That might sound like a lot, but it is really just a drop in the bucket compared to the annual $6.6 billion spent on pharmaceuticals for arthritis. Clearly, there are legions of ailing joints out in the world. The lower amount spent on glucosamine and chondroitin is partly related to their less frequent use, but primarily it reflects a more reasonable price compared to the patented pharmaceutical drugs.

In fact, the cost of these nutritional supplements has been dropping rapidly as numerous companies competing for consumer business have entered the marketplace. As an example, a one-month supply of a combination product supplying 1,500 mg of glucosamine sulfate and 1,200 mg of chondroitin sulfate is as little as $20 per month. And this is not an off-label bargain basement reject. This particular brand was independently tested for potency, as many brands have been. The monthly cost of taking glucosamine and/or chondroitin is quite reasonable in comparison to the cost of prescription osteoarthritis products. (A typical brand-name NSAID could cost up to $100 a month, or about $40 if it's a generic, but even this lower cost is double that of the natural glucosamine/chondroitin supplements.)

There's never been a better time to give glucosamine/chondroitin products a try to see if they will help your joints because product quality and cost are both the best they've ever been.

CHAPTER 4

How to Take Glucosamine and Chondroitin

By now it's clear that glucosamine and chondroitin get to the root of the problem: the joint, where they repair the damage caused by osteoarthritis. You are probably anxious to find out if you'll be among the majority of those with osteoarthritis who find relief with glucosamine and chondroitin. But you'll want to make sure you use these supplements in the best way—the way that has solid scientific research as a successful treatment for osteoarthritis behind it. That's what this chapter is all about. Here is where you'll find the nuts-and-bolts information on how to incorporate these supplements into your life.

Glucosamine Comes in Different Forms

Glucosamine is commonly available in three forms: glucosamine sulfate, glucosamine HCl, and N-acetyl glucosamine. The vast majority of the scientific research has used the glucosamine sulfate form. However, this does not mean the other forms of glucosamine are not effective. There are a few studies that have focused on the glucosamine HCl and N-acetyl glucosamine forms with promising results.

There are no studies comparing these glucos - amine forms to each other, so it is difficult to know if one is better than another. It would be prudent, if you had to choose only one, to stick with the glu-

Which glucosamine product is best?
There have not yet been any studies comparing the forms of glucosamine (glucosamine sulfate, glucosamine HCl, and N-acetyl glucosamine) to one another. For this reason, it is not yet known if one is more effective than another.

cosamine sulfate form since it has been the most thoroughly researched. However, there is also something to be said for hedging your bets by taking one of the combination products on the market which contain glucosamine sulfate, glucosamine HCl, and N-acetyl glucosamine.

Lower Weight Chondroitin Preferable

Unlike glucosamine, chondroitin is generally available in only one form: chondroitin sulfate. There are, however, varying weights of chondroitin sulfate and, as previously stated, the low-molecular-mass chondroitin is theoretically better absorbed. Chondroitin sulfate compounds differ slightly in terms of where the sulfate is attached to the chondroitin molecule and this difference in location accounts for the different weights of chondroitin sulfates (the lower weight chondroitin-4-sulfate and chondroitin-6-sulfate are the most plentiful chondroitin sulfates in the body).

Researchers have noted that the lower weight compounds are more easily absorbed, and are for this reason theoretically the preferred form. Some products on the market will specify on the label that the product contains "low-weight chondroitin sulfate."

Sulfate Plays a Role

It might be a good idea to make sure that there is at least some sulfate in the product you buy. In other words, including some glucosamine sulfate or chondroitin sulfate as opposed to only glucosamine HCl or N-acetyl glucosamine could be prudent.

There is some evidence that part of the reason why both glucosamine sulfate and chondroitin sulfate supplements aid joint health is because of the sulfate molecule they are attached to. Sulfate is a form of sulfur, and sulfur is an essential nutrient needed for the stabilization of the connective tissue matrix as well as for the manufacture of collagen. The idea that sulfur is needed for joint repair is nothing new. Back in 1934, a researcher first proposed that sulfur halts the degeneration of joints in those with arthritis.

When sulfate levels are low, the manufacture of new glycosaminoglycans (the complex compounds in the joint tissue, including chondroitin) is drastically stepped down, according to research in animals. In humans, it has been shown that a limited supply of sulfate also interferes with the production of new glycosaminoglycans.

Sulfate Needed for Healthy Cartilage

Sulfate (a component of glucosamine sulfate and chondroitin sulfate) is needed to build new cartilage. Taking the pain-reliever acetaminophen can lower sulfate levels in the body, further aggravating the malfunction of cartilage in osteoarthritic joints.

This slowing of glycosaminoglycan production can be a big problem for those with arthritis. Joints suffering from arthritis have an increased demand for glycosaminoglycans, so at the time when the joints are calling for more of these important compounds, they might not have enough sulfate available to produce them.

Glucosamine versus Chondroitin

Glucosamine and chondroitin play slightly different roles in joint tissue, but both have the end effect of rebuilding damaged cartilage. However, it is always reassuring to have a solid foundation in scientific research, and the simple fact is that glucosamine has been scrutinized in far more studies than chondroitin. This is not to say chondroitin doesn't work. It just means that glucosamine has been put under the microscope more often and in more people so, if you had to choose just one, for this reason glucosamine would be the better bet.

But why not hedge your bets and take a combination product? There are numerous products on the market today that contain a mixture of glucosamine and chondroitin. This way you'll be able to garner the benefits of both supplements.

Choosing to take a combination product has another, even more valuable benefit. Glucosamine and chondroitin have been found to have a synergistic benefit to the joints, rather than a simple additive effect which means that the total benefit exceeds that expected of each taken alone. This is because glycosaminoglycan production is being stimulated by the glucosamine while, at the same time, the chondroitin is inhibiting the breakdown of glycosaminoglycans. The net effect is the production of greater quantities of healthy cartilage.

> **Glucosamine and Chondroitin Work Synergistically**
> *Glucosamine and chondroitin taken together are more effective in joint recovery than either one used alone. In fact, they have a synergistic effect in slowing the progression of joint damage.*

For example, supplements of glucosamine HCl, low-molecular-weight chondroitin sulfate, and manganese ascorbate (a vitamin-mineral complex) were tested separately and in combination for how well they slowed cartilage degeneration in rabbits. While each of these supplements helped the rabbits a bit, when they were given as a combination product, the rabbits had the most joint protection. In the laboratory, petri dishes of cartilage show a much greater amount of new glycosaminoglycan growth when this same combination is given than when each of the components is used separately.

Who Should Consider Taking These Supplements?

The primary use of glucosamine and chondroitin is for the healing of joints addled with osteoarthritis damage. (Chapter 7 discusses additional health benefits of these supplements.) For this reason, adult men and women who have been diagnosed with osteoarthritis by a physician are the core group of people who should consider taking these supplements.

Even if your osteoarthritis is under control (either with the use of conventional NSAID medications or other means), you might want to consider taking glucosamine and chondroitin in order to prevent a future flare-up. However, there is no reason you can't wait until a flare-up starts before resuming, or commencing, the use of glucosamine and chondroitin.

Even people without any signs of osteoarthritis might consider these supplements. On each birthday after age sixty-five, you have a 2 percent greater risk of developing osteoarthritis. Thus, healthy older people might want to use glucosamine and chondroitin as insurance against developing osteoarthritis. This is particularly prudent "insurance" if you have other risk factors for osteoarthritis such as prior joint injuries, family history, or obesity.

Three Types Are "Right" for Taking Glucosamine/Chondroitin

1. *Adults with active cases of osteoarthrits—to restore joint health.*

2. *Adults with osteoarthritis that is currently under control—to reduce chances of relapse.*

3. *Healthy older people who are at risk for this disease—to lower the chances that it will ever develop.*

The Right Amount

Virtually all human research has uniformly used 1,500 mg of glucosamine per day, an amount that seems appropriate for most people. However, after taking this full amount of glucosamine for six to eight weeks, you could experiment to see if taking 1,000 mg per day, or even as little as 500 mg per day as a "maintenance" dose, will keep your symptoms at bay. The standard dose of chondroitin is 1,200 mg per day.

For example, Ray, a fifty-nine-year-old man with osteoarthritis of the knee, took 1,500 mg of glucosamine sulfate daily for several years and got significant relief from his knee discomfort. When he experimented with phasing out glucosamine altogether, his symptoms returned. Today, however, he is able to maintain the same level of relief that 1,500 mg per day initially provided by taking just 1,000 mg per day as a maintenance dose.

How much glucosamine and chondroitin should I take? *According to numerous research studies, a daily intake of 1,500 mg glucosamine and 1,200 mg chondroitin is an effective amount for most people.*

It is probably a good idea to start out at the recommended dosage of 1,500 mg per day, rather than experimenting with lower levels. Jeff, a thirty-five-year-old with osteoarthritis of the hip and knee as a result of sports injuries, had tried taking just 500 mg of glucosamine off and on for several months without significant pain relief.

After upping to the full 1,500 mg per day (along with 1,200 mg per day of chondroitin) and diligently taking it every day, he was able to start running again after having avoided that joint-jarring activity for the previous five years. He reports that his joints feel almost as good as in his younger years.

Once A Day Is All You Need

Taking glucosamine and chondroitin is more convenient than ever before. For starters, they are no longer sleepy, backwoods specialty supplements, they can now be found virtually everywhere: in natural foods stores, pharmacies, grocery stores, even warehouse discount stores.

In addition, glucosamine is easier than ever to

use. The original studies with this supplement used injections of glucosamine, a drawback because a medication that only comes in injectable form means people have to spend extra time and money at a physician's office. Fortunately glucosamine in pill form that was stable and well absorbed was developed. This original pill form was taken three times per day—500 mg each time, the standard recommendation—an improvement over injections, but still a hassle. Having to cart around your bottle of supplements all day, as well as remember to actually pop all three pills, was hard to do.

Now, research has found that taking 1,500 mg in one sitting is just as effective as the divided doses. You only have to remember once a day to take the supplement, and you can choose whichever time of day is most convenient for you.

The story is just about the same with chondroitin: it is also now known to be effective when taken once daily. In one study, chondroitin supplements were given one of two ways. In one method, 800 mg of chondroitin sulfate was provided to volunteers in one sitting. In the other method, 400 mg of chondroitin sulfate was given in the early part of the day and another 400 mg was given later in the day. Although both dosing schedules increased blood levels of the compounds associated with this supplement, the once-daily schedule resulted in higher levels.

Don't Give Up Too Soon

Don't expect instant relief after starting a regimen of glucosamine and/or chondroitin. Most research has found that these supplements need to be taken daily for at least four weeks in order to derive benefits. You should begin to experience increasing pain relief and increased mobility during this initial month, and many people continue to improve further in subsequent weeks and months.

A chart called a "Daily Pain Record" is a tool to help you track your pain on a day-to-day basis over a one-month period to determine how much, if at all, the glucosamine and/or chondroitin supplements are helping your osteoarthritis.

DAILY PAIN RECORD

DAY	PAIN LEVEL				
	0	1	2	3	4
1					
2					
3					
4					
5					
6					
7					
8					
9					
10					
11					
12					
13					
14					
15					
16					
17					
18					
19					
20					
21					
22					
23					
24					
25					
26					
27					
28					
29					
30					

What is your level of discomfort today?

0 None

1 Mild

2 Moderate

3
Moderately severe

4 Severe

Consider Cycling On and Off

After taking glucosamine and/or chondroitin for many months or years, you will have reached the peak of your pain relief with these supplements. At this point, it might be appropriate to lower your dosage to a maintenance dose. (For example, to 500–1,000 mg per day of glucosamine and/or 400–800 mg of chondroitin.) You might even be able to stop taking the supplements for a while.

The benefits of these supplements do not stop the day after you stop taking the pills. Several research studies have found that joint relief continues for many weeks, and sometimes up to three months after their use is discontinued. For this reason, some people have found that they can save money and the daily hassle of taking pills by using glucosamine and chondroitin on an intermittent basis.

Avoid Glucosamine Cream

Glucosamine and chondroitin should be used only in oral (pill) form for osteoarthritis. To date, there is no evidence that putting these compounds on the skin over a joint will provide any health benefit whatsoever, so it is probably a waste of money to use glucosamine or chondroitin in topical rub-on cream or gel forms.

The cream form, however, might have some merit for other health conditions. It has been favorably studied for relieving the itchiness of poison ivy and poison oak.

Will Glucosamine Work for You?

While study after study has shown glucosamine and chondroitin to have scientifically measurable benefits in the disease of osteoarthritis, there are no guarantees they will work in a particular individual's case. In general, however, clinical trials comparing glucosamine to a placebo found that glucosamine provided significant pain relief, joint mobility improvement, and other benefits in 52 to 55 percent of those taking it.

"Responders" Are in the Majority *More than half the people given glucosamine in clinical trials have a scientifically measurable improvement to their osteoarthritis.*

Researchers have identified a few criteria which influence who will be a "responder" (versus a non-responder) to supplemental therapy. Those with less severe cases (that is, mild-to-moderate cases of osteoarthritis) are more likely to respond to glucosamine. This makes sense, since the joints still have some amount of normally functioning cartilage that can be "jump-started" with the addition of glucosamine.

There have been reports that obesity hampers a person's response to glucosamine. But, it has yet to be tested whether simply increasing the glucosamine in such cases will overcome the less-than-ideal response.

In addition, there have also been anecdotal reports that people with active peptic ulcers and those taking diuretics are less likely to be among the glucosamine success stories. Again, the use of a "Daily Pain Record" chart can help you determine if you are a responder and if it is worth the trouble and expense to continue taking glucosamine and/or chondroitin.

Most Important of All, Start Early

It's just common sense: The earlier they are taken in the disease process, the more effective glucosamine and chondroitin are. Mild-to-moderate osteoarthritis has a good chance of being helped by these supplements. In the few studies that included patients with severe arthritis, their response was certainly less stellar than the response of those with more moderate cases of this disease. This is not to say, however, that you can't be helped if you have severe osteoarthritis. Try it, it's worth a test run.

Many people with osteoarthritis fail to seek help until years after symptoms begin. Be advised, though, that the sooner you start taking these supplements, the better your chances of reversing joint damage are.

CHAPTER 5

ADDITIONAL
JOINT PROTECTORS

Glucosamine and chondroitin are certainly in the frontlines when it comes to easing pain and healing joints damaged by osteoarthritis, but they are not necessarily the entire army. There are several other vitamins, minerals, and dietary supplements that serve as supporting soldiers to give your joints extra protection.

Low levels of several nutrients are associated with arthritis, although whether this is a cause or a result of arthritis is still a little murky. What is known is that joint pain and stiffness increase when a person is malnourished and symptoms improve when there is an increased intake of nutrients.

In addition, the inflammation common to arthritis can change the lining of the intestines, reducing the absorption of some nutrients, while at the same time increasing nutrient needs. Optimal intake of vitamins and minerals is also important to ensure that the body will have the building blocks necessary to rebuild joints and connective tissues damaged by an arthritis flare-up or by drug therapy.

Added Vitamins and Minerals Give Osteoarthritis a One-Two Punch

In numerous clinical trials, a combination of glucosa-mine and chondroitin has been shown to manage osteoarthritis, and vitamin C and manganese can support the action of these joint-healing supplements.

Vitamin C is certainly an important nutrient to consider as a supporting player for the health of your joints. The key story with this vitamin is that it is needed for collagen synthesis. In addition, it decreases free radical damage, which is one of the potential causes of osteoarthritis.

The mineral manganese also plays a supporting role in the body's manufacture of chondroitin. Although the role of manganese deficiency in the development of osteoarthritis has not yet been specifically researched, it is known that Western societies are at risk of suboptimal manganese intake.

In fact, approximately one in three Americans has low manganese intake. Why do we fall short with this mineral? For starters, modern farming techniques deplete manganese from the soil of farming lands and, in turn, from the food that is grown there. Furthermore, refined grains (white flour, white rice, and so on) are the predominant food choices in contemporary America and they contain only half the manganese of whole grains. It all adds up to a pretty suspicious situation.

Joint Disease Seen in Animals
In animals, manganese deficiency leads to cartilage problems and a form of joint disease. It has been suggested that the lack of this mineral in the diet, could cause the same problems in people.

Not surprisingly, there have already been several studies that use a combination of glucosamine, chondroitin, vitamin C, and manganese. In one clinical trial using this combination, symptoms of osteoarthritis in the knee were greatly reduced.

In another trial, published in the journal *Osteoarthritis and Cartilage*, ninety-three patients with osteoarthritis of the knee took this combination supplement or a placebo. Those with mild to moderate osteoarthritis who took the supplement showed significant improvement in their symptoms by the end of the six-month study. Those with severe osteoarthritis, however, showed fewer benefits. In an animal model, this same combination made it less likely that animals would even develop arthritis in the first place.

There are formulas on the market that contain the combination of glucosamine, chondroitin, vitamin C, and manganese. However, manganese can be "too much of a good thing." Concerns have been raised that some of these supplements contain excessive amounts of manganese which has prompted several manufacturers to reformulate their products with appropriate, lower amounts of manganese. (See Chapter 8 for more about manganese toxicity.)

Tips to "B" Healthier

Supplements of certain B vitamins may be just as effective in arthritis as NSAIDs—but without the side effects. In one study of B vitamins in arthritis, twenty-six men and women with osteoarthritis were given a combined supplement of folic acid and vitamin B_{12}, or a placebo, daily, for two months. During the study none of the patients used anti-arthritis drugs or any other supplements.

After taking the B-vitamin supplements for two months, the arthritis patients had better hand grip strength and less joint tenderness than those who were given a placebo. The beneficial effect was equivalent to that expected with NSAID use. The researcher of this study summed up the benefits of B-vitamin supplements over conventional drugs in the *Journal of the American College of Nutrition:* "Side effects with the vitamin combination were none; side effects of NSAID are many, and the cost of vit - amins . . . is lower."

Niacinamide is a form of vitamin B_3. Several decades ago, this form of vitamin B_3 was first reported in the *Journal of the American Geriatric Society* to provide dramatic improvement for those with osteoarthritis, in terms of joint mobility, inflammation, and pain. This original research indicated it might take up to a month to see benefits, but then the improvements would continue for many years while niacinamide was taken. This early research administered 500 mg of niacinamide three to four times per day.

It's taken a long time, but researchers have finally resumed studies with this vitamin. In a recent double-blind study, the benefits originally reported with niacinamide were supported in seventy-two patients with osteoarthritis. Researchers found that niacinamide produced a 29 percent improvement in all symptoms and signs compared to a 10 percent worsening in the placebo group.

Niacinamide is generally well tolerated and without side effects. Unlike niacin (another form of vitamin B_3), niacinamide does not produce flushing of the skin. However, with the amounts used for arthritis, it is prudent to have blood tests several times a year to monitor for any possible liver damage.

Be Careful with Niacinamide
Although niacinamide is generally safe to use, it can cause serious liver- damage problems for a few people. Work with your doctor if you are taking more than 1,500 mg per day.

Not surprisingly then, this supplement should not be used by anyone with pre-existing liver disease. In addition, people with diabetes need to know that niacinamide might alter requirements for insulin. Thus, you should work with your health care provider to monitor blood-sugar levels and adjust your medication, as needed. Since the B vitamins are known to work better as a unit than when taken individually, it is advisable to take a B-complex supplement along with these individual Bs.

Vitamin D Fits the Bill for Prevention

For anyone with osteoarthritis, a low intake of vitamin D is like adding insult to injury. Worsening knee problems are two to four times more likely in vitamin D–deficient osteoarthritics. In another study, people with low blood levels of vitamin D were found more likely to develop osteoarthritis of the hip.

Foods rich in vitamin D, sun exposure, or vitamin D supplements appear to be equally effective in raising the levels of vitamin D enough to hamper the progression of the disease. However, keep in mind that supplementation with vitamin D should be limited to 200–400 mg per day since this vitamin can be toxic in higher amounts.

Fighting Free Radicals

The antioxidant nutrients are particularly important for anyone with arthritis. The inflammatory process causes large numbers of harmful compounds called free radicals to be released. A free radical is missing a vital part of itself—one of its electrons. In an effort to restore the balance of a paired electron, it reacts with any nearby molecule in the body, such as fats, proteins, or even DNA.

The end result is a deadly game of hot potato. As the original free radical passes off its unpaired electron or steals an electron from another molecule, that molecule becomes unbalanced. This newly formed free radical then interacts with yet another molecule in pursuit of stability, and so on. Essentially, antioxidants act as a referee in the body, ending the potentially out-of-hand game of free-radical hot potato that, if left unchecked, can destroy the body.

Vitamin E is an important antioxidant in the body's defenses against free radicals. In one study, patients with osteoarthritis took 600 mg of vitamin E per day, or a placebo, for ten days. Later, they

Antioxidants: The Electron Donors
Antioxidants have the unique ability to donate the much-sought-after electron that free radicals need without becoming free radicals themselves.

switched to the opposite treatment of either vitamin E or the placebo. A little more than half of those taking vitamin E experienced pain reduction, while only 4 percent of the placebo group could say the same. In other research, vitamin E was compared to the NSAID diclofenac and was shown to be just as effective as that medication for increasing joint mobility and improving walking time.

Dr. Timothy McAlindon at the Arthritis Center, Boston University Medical Center has been studying the protective role of antioxidant nutrients in osteoarthritis. Of the 640 participants in his Framingham Osteoarthritis Cohort study, a higher intake of vitamin C, another antioxidant, was related to a three-fold lesser risk of disease progression. The benefits of vitamin C were seen in both men and women, at various stages of disease severity, and in both users and non-users of supplements. The benefits of beta-carotene and vitamin E were not as strong in this study.

Dr. McAlindon notes that ". . . the effect of vitamin C appeared stronger and more consistent than that of beta carotene or of vitamin E." This may be explained by the watery environment of certain parts of the joint that would benefit more from a water-soluble, rather than a fat-soluble, antioxidant. (Vitamin C is water-soluble, while vitamin E and beta-carotene are fat-soluable.)

Dr. McAlindon summed up his research by stating that a "high intake of antioxidant micronutrients, especially vitamin C, may reduce the risk of cartilage loss and disease progression in people with [osteoarthritis]."

There are many antioxidant nutrients, but the

ones with documented success in arthritis are vitamin C, vitamin E, and selenium. However, the bioflavonoids, such as quercitin, and the proanthocyanidins in pine bark and grapeseed extract may also be helpful in preventing accumulation of fluids, swelling, and pain in the joints.

The Latest Aids: SAMe and MSM

S-adenosylmethionine (SAMe), which is related to the amino acid methionine, holds a lot of promise for folks with osteoarthritis. While this supplement was being investigated as a treatment for depression, many of the depressed patients who also happened to have osteoarthritis began to report to their doctors that SAMe was giving them relief from their joint troubles.

Since then, several large trials have examined the role of SAMe in osteoarthritis. In the more than 22,000 patients who have now been treated with SAMe in trials, it is clear that SAMe is at least as effective as NSAIDs, according to a review published in the *Alternative Medicine Reviews*. The studies have generally provided 400–1,200 mg per day of SAMe.

SAMe is formed in the body by combining the essential amino acid methionine with adenosyltri-phosphate (ATP). SAMe is involved in dozens of biochemical reactions in the body, and works with several B vitamins to support certain body functions. More importantly, this compound is needed for the body to make cartilage components such as chondroitin sulfate. When the body has a deficiency of SAMe, the joints are less able to maintain their springy, resilient qualities.

SAMe is generally without side effects, although gastrointestinal disturbances and nausea have been occasionally reported. If you have bipolar disorder or Parkinson's disease, you shouldn't take this supplement.

Methylsulfonylmethane (MSM) has recently become popular as a pain reliever for
those with arthritis. MSM is related
to DMSO—the topically applied
substance which saw its heyday in
the 1960s and 1970s. Unfortunately, DMSO is associated with many
side effects, such as blistering, diarrhea, dizziness, nausea, and rashes,
and should be used cautiously.

The Cartilage Builder
SAMe is yet another of the important building blocks needed to make new crops of healthy, strong cartilage.

In contrast, MSM—which is taken orally—has
been shown in some research to ease the pain and
inflammation of joints without the side effects of
DMSO. Animal research suggests that MSM protects against the breakdown of cartilage in joints.
MSM (as well as DMSO) is believed to aid in arthritis
through its sulfur content, a mineral that is needed
for a wide array of body functions.

Joint tissues need sulfur to help stabilize the connective tissue matrix. Research dating back almost
a century had indicated that people with arthritis are
more likely to be deficient in sulfur. While this is intriguing, there have thus far only been anecdotal
claims for MSM as an arthritis treatment; the hard
scientific research remains to be done. However,
this supplement is safe and you can try one to three
grams daily to see if your symptoms would be improved.

Herbal Relief

Cayenne peppers, plants native to Central America,
have become one of the hottest arthritis treatments
around. Capsaicin—the active ingredient in cayenne
peppers—is applied topically as a cream and reduces the pain of arthritis by depleting the nerves
of "substance P," a chemical that carries pain sen-
sations to the brain. Topical creams which contain
0.025 percent capsaicin cream are generally used

four times per day. They are widely available in health food stores, drug stores, etc.

Initially, capsaicin might cause a burning sensation, but this discomfort quickly goes away—as (in many cases) does the arthritis pain. A word of caution: wash your hands after applying capsaicin cream, as it can be painful and irritating if any residual cream on your hands comes into contact with your eyes or other sensitive tissues.

Pain, Pain Go Away
The hot cayenne pepper, well known for its role in the kitchen, also has a role in your medicine chest. Creams made from cayenne can provide relief from joint pain.

The Devil's claw plant (*Harpagophytum pricumbens*) was given this vivid name in reference to the claw-shaped growths—complete with imposing thorns adorned with several fingerlike growths—which wrap around and protect the plant's seeds. The underground tubers of this plant were used medicinally by indigenous African tribes, primarily for arthritis conditions.

Europeans traveling to Africa heard tales of the health-enhancing properties of Devil's claw and brought samples of it back to Germany and other European countries to test. The clinical research using Devil's claw root for arthritis conditions proved favorable and Devil's claw quickly gained recognition throughout Europe for alleviating arthritis symptoms, particularly for reducing pain and inflammation. More research with this herb is warranted, but you could give it a try if you haven't been able to find adequate pain relief with other methods.

Ginger, a popular food spice, has been used as a folk medicine for numerous maladies. Ginger holds an important place in several traditional systems of medicine. When researchers put ginger to the test in both rheumatoid arthritis and osteoarthritis cases, more than three-quarters of those tested experienced relief from pain and swelling.

Boswellia serrata, an herb from the Ayurvedic tradition, improves blood supply to the joints and prevents tissue deterioration. Boswellia is valuable because, although it acts like a NSAID, it does not produce the side effects of pharmaceutical NSAIDs. One clinical trial of 175 rheumatoid arthritis patients found that Boswellic acid supplements (the active ingredient in *Boswellia serrata*), improved grip strength, morning pain and stiffness, and physical performance in 97 percent of patients after three to four weeks of treatment.

The turmeric plant has long been used in India as a source of spice and clothing dye. Today, *curcumin*—an extract from the turmeric spice—is gaining worldwide recognition for its potent ability to quell inflammation. (As one of the oldest anti-inflammatory drugs used by traditional Indian medicine, turmeric is not actually a new discovery.) Animal studies, as well as some preliminary work with people, show promising results.

Beware of Nightshade Vegetables

Could your arthritis symptoms be traced back to what is served on your dinner plate? It's possible if you are eating foods from the nightshade family. In the 1960s, Dr. Norman Childers, a horticulturist from New Jersey's Rutgers University, noticed a worsening of his own arthritis pain and stiffness after eating vegetables from the nightshade class, and an easing of his symptoms when he avoided these foods.

Since Dr. Childers' discovery, the role of nightshade plants in arthritis has been a topic of heated controversy. While many with arthritis give testimony about the strong relationship they have experienced between nightshade plants and joint problems, the scientific community has yet to back up these claims. Various alkaloids found in night-shade plants, such as atropine, nicotine, and scopo-lamine, have been hypothesized to provoke arthritis symptoms.

Reports vary widely (from five to 66 percent) on the number of people sensitive to nightshade plants. In order to determine if you are among those affected by this class of foods, simply eliminate nightshade plants from your diet. If you are sensitive, it may take up to six weeks to notice a beneficial effect from avoiding these plants.

The Nightshade Family

Nightshade vegetables include bell peppers, egg-plant, paprika, potatoes (but not sweet potatoes or yams), and tomatoes. Tobacco is also in this family of plants.

Hot and Cold Relief

Diathermy or "deep heat" has been reported as a valuable aid for controlling pain and increasing joint mobility in arthritis. It is administered by high frequency sound waves (ultrasound) or electro-mechanical irradiation (microwave or short wave). The application of heat is thought to increase the pain threshold and relieve pain by reducing nerve-conduction velocity. On the downside, diathermy can be expensive and time consuming.

In recent years, there have been only two randomized clinical trials that assessed the effectiveness of diathermy. Both involved patients with osteo-arthritis of the knee, and after the diathermy treatments there were only slight improvements which were not great enough to reach statistical significance.

Play It Smart with Heat Therapy

Heat can be very soothing, but don't apply heat to a joint that is already hot and swollen, or continue heat treatment for more than about thirty minutes.

For now, therefore, it would seem that this therapy does not provide effective arthritis treatment.

Other forms of locally applied heat, such as a

heating pad, hot water bottle, or heat lamps, are valued by many with arthritis for the comfort they provide. Heating the skin increases blood circulation and helps the muscles relax.

Best of Both Worlds
Some people with arthritis find it helpful to alternate heat and cold to maximize the benefits of both.

Some people with arthritis consider the opposite treatment—cold therapy or cryotherapy—effective. Cold therapy is conducted by applying gel-filled, refreezable cold packs or plastic bags filled with ice to the joint, making sure to protect the skin with a layer of cloth, and to limit the treatment to twenty minutes every few hours. This therapy is fairly effective in reducing inflammation.

Hydrotherapy, in baths, spas, springs, tanks, or tubs, is one of the oldest and most enjoyable forms of medical treatment. Although its effects are temporary, they are pleasant and pain relieving. Hydrotherapy basically works by acting as a whole-body heat treatment, warming all the joints at once to ease both pain and stiffness (although it has no effect on inflammation, and heat is not recommended if there is inflammation).

Could Needles Relieve Pain, Instead of Causing It?

Tap Into Your Natural Painkillers
Modern research suggests that acupuncture relieves the pain of arthritis and other conditions by causing the release of endorphins (the body's natural morphine) which act as natural painkillers.

Acupuncture is a 2,000-year-old branch of Chinese medicine based on the belief that life force (called *Chi*) flows through the body along meridians or channels. Blockage of these meridians leads to ill health, while opening the meridians with the use of needles inserted into the skin restores health. In fact, acupuncture is becoming an increasingly common and effective treatment for osteoarthritis.

A group of people waiting for a total hip replacement agreed to take part in a study. Half were treated with acupuncture, and the other half were given advice and a set of hip exercises. Over the eight-week study, the acupuncture group showed significant improvement, while the other group experienced no changes.

Other research has documented that real acupuncture, as opposed to sham acupuncture (where needles are inserted in sites not believed to have any health benefit) is more effective for pain relief of knee osteoarthritis than the sham treatment which is equivalent to a placebo. Thus, this study shows that acupuncture has merit for use in osteoarthritis. Additional research found that acupuncture treatment in thirty-two osteoarthritis patients treated twice weekly for three weeks improved pain by 23 percent and mobility by 28 percent.

CHAPTER 6

USING SUPPLEMENTS AND CONVENTIONAL MEDICINES

The arthritis-drug market is the source of big bucks for the pharmaceutical industry. These drugs bring in $6.6 billion per year, and this astounding number doesn't even include such standards in arthritis relief such as acetaminophen.

With all that money pouring into the pharmaceutical coffers, one would expect osteoarthritis patients to feel great. But the sad fact is that even though they're spending all that money on arthritis drugs, many patients do not get satisfactory relief from their pain and disability. Adding insult to injury, conventional arthritis drugs tend to come with an additional steep price: that of undesirable side effects.

Glucosamine and chondroitin are great, side-effect-free options to explore in place of conventional drugs. But you don't necessarily have to choose one over the other. There's no reason you can't maximize your osteoarthritis relief by taking a combination of both glucosamine/chondroitin and conventional arthritis drugs such as NSAIDs.

Conventional Treatments Fall Short

Although magazines and television are overflowing with ads for over-the-counter and prescription drugs for arthritis, the truth is that conventional medicine continues to fail in their search for a cure to arthritis. Instead they merely offer pain-killing medications that only mask the problem (and come with a hefty price in side effects).

Aspirin is the most basic of anti-inflammatory drugs used to combat arthritis. The easing of the inflammation combined with its analgesic quality has made this the drug of choice for many people. Aspirin is a relatively inexpensive drug, but what it offers in reasonable pricing, it makes up for in harmful side effects which can include headaches, nausea, ringing in the ears, and/or stomach pain,.

Nonsteroidal anti-inflammatory drugs (NSAIDs) are used in cases where aspirin is unsuitable. NSAIDs, which include ibuprofen (Motrin), indomethacin (Indocin), fenoprofen (Nalfon), naproxen (Alleve), sulindac (Clinoril), tolmetin (Tolectin), and many others, are less likely than aspirin to cause stomach upset but have other harmful side effects. Newer generations of NSAIDs, such as celecoxib (Celebrex) and rofecoxib (Vioxx), have entered the market, but even these are not without problems.

NSAIDs Have a Dark Side
Nonsteroidal anti-inflammatory drugs (NSAIDs) are commonly used by those with arthritis, but they all too often cause side effects, such as stomach upset and ulcers.

NSAIDs act as painkillers while also reducing inflammation in the joints and soft tissues; they do not, however, cure or halt the progress of the disease. Their mechanism of action is to block the production of prostaglandins (hormone-like substances in the body that can produce inflammation and pain). The list of adverse effects from NSAIDs is numerous, and in some cases very severe, but the most common side effects are diarrhea, indigestion, nausea, and peptic ulcer.

Corticosteroids act similarly to natural hormones in order to suppress inflammation. However, since inflammation is a necessary process for the body's immune defense system, corticosteroids can impair the body's ability to deal with infections and injuries. These drugs may also suppress activity of the adrenal cortex. Corticosteroids are best used on a short-term basis.

Penicillamine, a synthetic derivative of penicillin, is another conventional treatment for arthritis. As with other conventional treatments, penicillamine can result in serious side effects, including bleeding, gastrointestinal upset, and liver problems.

Artificial Joints: Are They the Answer?

One other option of conventional medicine: radical surgery in which an artificial joint takes the place of the problematic joint. Even this extreme step is not a cure, since the artificial joint has a lifespan of only about ten years, when the surgery will have to be repeated. (Although there are exceptions, especially with cementless hip replacements where bone and metal fuse.) Despite the generally limited lifespan of artificial joints, lots of people with arthritis are going under the knife when their symptoms become so severe they feel there is no other option.

Joint Replacements Are Common Procedure
Each year, about 267,000 knee replacements and 168,000 artificial hip surgeries are performed.

A Closer Look at Pain Relievers

As previously stated, NSAIDs work by blocking the production of prostaglandins (hormonelike substances that can trigger inflammation). But blocking these inflammation-promoting prostaglandins is also the source of NSAIDs' side effects. Prosta-glandins play other roles in the body, for example they are needed to control the secretion of gastric juices and the mucus that serves as stomach lining. This is why NSAIDs are linked to ulcers and even life-

NSAIDs Have High Costs in Many Ways

Not only are NSAID medications expensive, they also lead to costly treatment of their side effects. Each year, $2 billion is spent to treat the side effects of NSAIDs.

threatening gastric bleeding when used long-term.

NSAIDs cause some disturbing side effects, ranging from indigestion and gastrointestinal hemorrhage to kidney failure. These side effects are serious business, with the NSAID-induced hemorrhages leading to at least 103,000 hospitalizations each year and 16,500 deaths.

And there is even worse news about standard drugs used for osteoarthritis pain. Aspirin and NSAIDs not only inhibit the repair of cartilage, they actually accelerate cartilage destruction. This means that, over time, aspirin and NSAIDs might actually worsen the disease they are "treating." In other words, although aspirin and NSAIDs might suppress symptoms, they also speed up the progression of the disease—not a worthwhile trade-off.

Ironically, NSAIDs Worsen Osteoarthritis

NSAIDs, which are taken to relieve osteoarthritis symptoms, have been documented to actually accelerate joint damage.

Cox-2 inhibitors (for example, Celebrex and Vioxx) were thought of as a breakthrough in improved arthritis treatment when they emerged on the market in 1999 because they target the specific prostaglandins that trigger inflammation, and don't affect those that play a role in stomach juices and mucus lining. However, the Cox-2 drugs come with a steep price tag ($3 to $6 per day) and, just recently, reports of a scary risk of side effects.

In the *Journal of the American Medical Association*, a leading cardiologist reported that Celebrex and Vioxx have a connection to heart problems. Specifically, these arthritis drugs could cause a small increase in heart attacks and ischemic strokes, a type of stroke. The cardiologist speculates that this risk is related to the drugs promoting the formation of blood clots.

While this new risk with Cox-2 drugs still requires further study to confirm, it leads one to wonder why anyone would take the unnecessary risk of putting their heart in jeopardy when there are safer, more effective, and cheaper alternatives such as glucosamine and chondroitin. Anyone with a personal or family history of heart disease should be especially careful of the risk that Cox-2 drugs might pose to cardiovascular health.

Glucosamine Works Better Than Conventional Medicine

Numerous head-to-head studies show that glucosamine is as effective as ibuprofen for symptomatic relief of osteoarthritis. For example, a group of 200 people with osteoarthritis of the knee agreed to take part in a one-month study. Half took 1,500 mg of glucosamine daily, and the other half took 1,200 mg of ibuprofen daily. Symptoms, including pain at night, pain after immobility, after standing, and after getting up from a chair, as well as walking distance and limitation of daily living activities, were recorded as a single score on the Lequesne index.

At the start of the study, the average Lequesne score for each group was sixteen. By the end of the study, both groups had dropped six points. In other words, the glucosamine was just as effective as the drug treatment.

Lequesne Index

The Lequesne index is a tool used in medical research to measure the severity of osteoarthritis symptoms. By combining the answers to a series of questions about ability to use a joint, pain, and range of motion, a single score is obtained.

Glucosamine Goes Head-to-Head with NSAIDs

When glucosamine and chondroitin are compared to NSAID medications, the natural supplements show that they pass muster in terms of effectively easing osteoarthritis symptoms.

The story is the same with chondroitin. Chondroitin sulfate (1,200 mg per day) was compared to 50 mg daily of the NSAID diclofenac (Voltaren). The Lequesne score dropped 78 percent with chondroitin, and 63 percent with diclofenac. When chondroitin was compared to ibuprofen (both groups took 1,200 mg daily), the chondroitin proved more effective in relieving symptoms.

It really makes sense to choose glucosamine and/or chondroitin instead of NSAIDs. You should get the same relief, and you'll skip the side effects.

Slow and Steady Wins the Race

The research is clear and unequivocal that glucosamine and chondroitin are just as effective as NSAIDs for symptomatic relief in osteoarthritis. However, there is a caveat. These supplements have a lag time before benefits are noted, whereas the NSAIDs are pretty much immediately effective.

For instance, in the glucosamine/ibuprofen study discussed earlier, 48 percent of the ibuprofen patients responded in the first week, but only 28 percent of the glucosamine group responded that quickly. By the end of the study, the numbers were neck and neck. Glucosamine and chondroitin take longer to work, but the wait is worth it.

Lessen Your Use of NSAIDs

A handful of studies have provided osteoarthritis patients with either glucosamine or chondroitin, and then let them continue to take their NSAID medication, as needed, for optimal pain relief. Without fail, these studies report that the need for NSAIDs drops with time. For instance, in one such study supplying 800 mg of chondroitin sulfate to those with osteoarthritis of the finger joints, hip, and/or knee, the amount of NSAIDs required to relieve pain was reduced by an impressive 72 percent.

In another study, also based on chondroitin supplements, NSAID use was allowed for severe pain. By the end of the trial, the patients took an average of 2.4 tablets of NSAIDs per month, whereas the placebo group was taking an average of 7.6 tablets.

The effect of glucosamine on inflammation has also been compared to NSAIDs. Remember that the main thing NSAIDs do is reduce inflammation. In an animal model, a combination of glucosamine and NSAIDs is best at reducing inflammation. In fact, this combination allowed the researchers to lower the NSAID dose two to three times and still retain the same amount of inflammation relief.

This means that even if you aren't able to entirely eliminate your use of NSAIDs, at least you will have lessened your risk for NSAID-related side effects by using fewer of these drugs.

Integrative Medicine Makes Sense

Integrative medicine is based on the philosophy of using what works best for a patient, whether that is conventional or alternative medicine. For the case of osteoarthritis, integrative medicine might mean, for some people, supplementing with glucosamine/chondroitin and continuing to take a small amount of NSAID medications.

Synergy of Treatment

The mechanism by which glucosamine/chondroitin quells inflammation in the body is different than that for NSAIDs. For this reason, some experts have suggested that the combined use of glucosamine/chondroitin with NSAIDs might have a synergistic effect as anti-inflammatory agents.

The idea here is that glucosamine/chondroitin

and NSAIDs, when taken at the same time, each contributes to easing inflammation in its own way. And the net effect is that inflammation vanishes from a swollen joint.

Try Glucosamine and Chondroitin Alone

Synergy Gives More "Bang for the Buck" than Expected

Synergy is the concept that two substances, when used together, provide more benefit than when either was used individually.

There have been many examples in this chapter about how glucosamine and/or chondroitin supplements can work alongside NSAID medications. Even so, from a holistic health standpoint, it makes the most sense to try these supplements alone—that is, without the NSAIDs. NSAIDs always come with a risk of side effects.

If you can possibly cut NSAIDs out of your life, you'll be the better for it. However, that is not a realistic goal for some severe cases of osteoarthritis. In such cases, reducing reliance on NSAIDs would be the next best thing.

CHAPTER 7

OSTEOARTHRITIS AND BEYOND

The lion's share of the research and attention about glucosamine and chondroitin is focused on osteoarthritis. But these supplements have other roles in health. Chances are, you started taking glucosamine or chondroitin for your stiff knee or achy hip, but did you know that your cholesterol levels might be dropping at the same time, and that your spouse may sleep better because you're not snoring? Let's look at the other benefits of glucosamine and chondroitin.

Atherosclerosis

Cardiovascular diseases claim the lives of almost one million Americans each year, more than any other disease. One in five Americans will eventually develop some form of cardiovascular disease. Although the initiation and progression of heart disease is a complex, multifaceted process, most research agrees that elevated cholesterol levels are a major contributor, since cholesterol is closely linked to the development of arteriosclerosis. Arteriosclerosis—commonly known as "hardening of the arteries"—occurs when the walls of the arteries lose their elasticity, thus interfering with proper circulation.

Atherosclerosis is the most common type of arteriosclerosis. With atherosclerosis, the hardening is a result of a buildup of fatty deposits. Athero -

sclerotic arteries are hard, inflexible, clogged with clumps of cholesterol, and more likely to develop high blood pressure. Even worse, when the coronary arteries (which feed the heart) are clogged, then the situation is known as coronary artery disease and the stage is set for a heart attack.

Tracking Your Cholesterol Numbers

The total cholesterol level generally deemed a low risk for heart disease is below 200 milligrams per deciliter of blood. If yours is above 240 mg/dl, there is cause for alarm.

Chondroitin sulfate has a documented role in protecting the health of blood vessels. Although the focus of this book is on the role chondroitin plays in the joints, it is also found in the lining of the blood vessels where it helps prevent the movement of blood across the blood vessel lining, inhibits the clumping of blood platelets, and lowers blood cholesterol levels.

In all these roles, chondroitin contributes to healthier circulation and a lower risk of heart disease. Research has found that chondroitin does, indeed, prevent atherosclerosis in animals and humans, and further lowers the chances of a heart attack in people who already have the disease.

If you're taking chondroitin for an achy joint, it's nice to know that your heart might garner a little protection as well.

Dry Eyes

If your tear ducts don't make enough tears to keep your eyes moist, they can feel continually dry and irritated, with a burning, itchy sensation. Dry eyes are more common in women, especially after menopause. They can even be a symptom of a serious health problem, such as rheumatoid arthritis or lupus, or a side effect of medication.

Artificial tears are a common way to relieve symptoms. And there is research showing that the inclusion of chondroitin sulfate in artificial tear products can improve their ability to lessen the feelings of burning, itching and foreign body sensation. Chondroitin sulfate is not yet commercially available in artificial tear products, but it should be in the not-too-distant future.

Kidney Stones

Kidney stones, which are much more common in Western countries, can be formed when substances in urine, such as calcium, precipitate into stones, calcium oxalate stones being the most common type. Kidney stones result in severe pain, accompanied by chills, fever, and nausea.

Chondroitin can lend a hand since it is naturally present in the urinary system, in such places as the bladder wall lining. One study reports that oral administration of glycosaminoglycans (chondroitin and related compounds) lowers urinary oxalate levels in individuals prone to accumulating oxalates, and lower oxalate levels are presumed to result in fewer kidney stones.

Avoiding New Kidney Stones
To help reduce your chances of forming new kidney stones if you are prone to them, make sure you drink plenty of water, eat a high-fiber diet, minimize your intake of animal proteins, and avoid chocolate, spinach, and rhubarb (all sources of oxalate).

Migraine

Migraines are a regular occurrence for 26 million Americans. These intense headaches are triggered by disturbances of the blood vessels in the head and, on average, last more than seventeen hours. There is an intriguing case report in the medical literature about glucosamine and migraines. It seems that a frequent migraine sufferer was taking glucosamine for osteoarthritis, and in the course of that treatment, the patient's migraines stopped.

To ascertain whether this was a real benefit of glucosamine, or simply a coincidence, ten volunteers who regularly faced migraines were asked to take glucosamine supplements daily. After a four-to-six week period in which no major changes were noted, the volunteers started to report a substantial drop in the frequency and/or intensity of their headaches. Glucosamine's role in blood-vessel-health is hypothesized to be the source of its benefits for migraine.

Snoring

There is an interesting study where chondroitin sulfate was sprayed into the noses of chronic snorers. Because chondroitin sulfate forms a coating on the nasal passages, this is thought to curtail snoring. The study found that it did indeed help—the snorers only snored for two-thirds of their usual snoring time. It is not yet known if oral (pill) forms of chondroitin would provide this same benefit.

TMJ

Temporomandibular joint syndrome (TMJ) is a disorder of the joint in the jaw bone. Chronic neck pain, headaches, "popping" noises when using the jaw, toothaches, and overall pain are the hallmark symptoms of TMJ. The cause of TMJ is often traced to clenching the jaw muscles and tooth grinding, behaviors which, in turn, exert pressure on the jaw joint and can wear down the cartilage there, essentially leading to osteoarthritis in that joint.

There is a report of fifty TMJ patients who were treat-

Simple TMJ Test
To see if you might have TMJ, simply put your little fingers in your ears and press forward. Then, open and close your mouth. If you hear a clicking noise and feel your jawbone push against your fingers, you might have TMJ and should consult a health professional.

ed with either glucosamine or a mixture of chondroitin and vitamin C. An impressive 80 percent of these patients responded to the treatment with a reduction in joint noises, pain, and swelling. These benefits were evident within the first two weeks of the study.

In another study, forty-five TMJ patients were randomly assigned to take either glucosamine or ibuprofen over a three-month period for their TMJ symptoms. Three-quarters of the glucosamine group responded to the treatment, while only 61 percent of the ibuprofen group improved. When the patients who responded to either treatment were examined more closely, it was found that the glucosamine led to a significantly greater pain reduction than the ibuprofen.

Ulcers

Stomach ulcers are a common problem, affecting one out of every ten people in their lifetime. Stomach ulcers (technically known as peptic ulcers) are caused when the mucous membrane of the stomach or upper portion of the intestines become eroded, and are worsened by the constant exposure to acidic stomach juices in the eroded area. NSAID medications irritate the protective mucous membranes, setting the stage for ulcers which cause burning pain and sometimes nausea.

When osteoarthritis patients are able to toss out their NSAID medications in favor of glucosamine, they are at lower risk for ulcers since the ulcer-promoting NSAIDs are no longer in their system. If you are even able to reduce your reliance on NSAIDs by using glucosamine, your stomach stands to benefit. Glucosamine, unlike NSAIDs, does not irritate the GI tract, and it has another benefit: glucosamine stimulates the production of protective gastric mucus which could potentially bolster the stomach's resistance to ulcers.

Wound Healing

The healing of wounds requires, among other things, the raw materials to make replacement skin and other soft tissues. Glucosamine and chondroitin both qualify as such raw materials. Laboratory studies on animals and humans all document that glucosamine and chondroitin promote improved healing of wounds.

CHAPTER 8

SAFETY
PROFILE

Glucosamine and chondroitin are made by the body for use in several locations, including the joints. This bodes well for their safety profile because compounds that are not foreign to the body are less likely to cause problems, and this certainly seems to be the case with glucosamine and chondroitin. Even so, there are a handful of safety concerns to consider, particularly if you have shellfish allergies or a sensitive stomach.

Chondroitin might have a mild blood-thinning effect, and for this reason people taking anticoagulant (blood-thinning) drugs should use this supplement with caution, or better yet use a product containing only glucosamine which does not have this effect.

It's a relief to know that glucosamine and chondroitin supplements have been safely used in osteoarthritis patients with other health problems, such as circulatory disease, depression, diabetes, liver disorders, and lung disorders. In all these cases, the glucosamine and chondroitin supplementation for osteoarthritis did not interfere with the course or treatment of those other conditions.

Slight Stomach Upset Most Common Problem

All the clinical trials of glucosamine and chondroitin include reports on side effects and, in study after study, the research has consistently documented the safety and tolerability of these supplements. For instance, in one study evaluating the tolerability of glucosamine in 1,208 patients, 88 percent of those taking this supplement reported absolutely no side effects. Of the side effects reported by the other 12 percent, all of them were mild. Most common was the approximately 3 to 5 percent of people who reported diarrhea, heartburn, nausea, and/or stomach upset, a finding that is consistent with the adverse events reported in other studies. Similarly, with chondroitin about 3 percent of users report nausea or stomach upset.

Side Effects Uncommon, but Do Occur

Aside from stomach upsets, other problems have been reported by an extremely small number of users (less than one percent). These include constipation, drowsiness, edema, head - ache, insomnia, and skin reactions.

Keep in mind that this slight risk of GI upset is still much lower than the risk of stomach problems seen with the use of NSAIDs. In fact, in one animal model, the researchers found that the toxicity of glucosamine compared to the NSAID indometacin was ten to thirty times more favorable for the glucosamine than for the NSAID.

Diabetics Can Rest Assured

For a while, the safety of glucosamine supplements for people with diabetes came into question. Some rat studies had found that the continuous administration of high doses of intravenous glucosamine led to insulin resistance. However, these very high levels of glucosamine are vastly different from the standard low doses of glucosamine pills taken by people.

The definitive word in glucosamine's safety for those with diabetes came from a large, three-year placebo-controlled study of glucosamine. This study carries much more weight than the rat studies since, for starters, it is actually with people instead of animals. In addition, the long duration of this study is another mark in its favor. In this study, people taking standard doses of glucosamine did not show any increases in blood-sugar levels. In fact, the opposite was true. There was actually a slight decrease in fasting-blood-sugar levels in the glu- cosamine users, compared to the placebo group's levels.

Understanding Insulin Resistance

Insulin is a hormone needed to regulate levels of sugar in the blood. When the body is resistant to insulin, blood-sugar levels can increase and interfere with normal body functions.

And, when analyzed separately, patients who entered the study with baseline blood-sugar levels that were higher than normal showed a tendency for their blood sugar to drop while taking glucosamine.

If you have diabetes and want to be completely safe while taking glucosamine supplements, simply increase your blood-sugar monitoring. If you notice any elevation, stop taking the supplement and see if your blood sugar then drops.

Mind Your Minerals

There have been reports that some glucosamine supplements contain too much manganese, a mineral generally found in com- bination products as manganese ascorbate. Although there have been no symptoms of manga - nese toxicity reported by any studies, there is a theoretical risk.

Signs of Too Much Manganese

Manganese toxicity can cause coughs, hypertension, iron- deficiency anemia neurological problems, tremor, and weakness.

The Tolerable Upper Intake Level for manganese, established by the National Academy of Sciences' Institute of Medicine, is 11 mg per day. In a 2001 study, some glucosamine supplements were found to provide up to 30 mg per dosage. Fortunately, in light of the newly established Tolerable Upper Intake Level for manganese, many manufacturers are reformulating their products to be within recommended levels, and this is unlikely to be a problem in the future.

As an interesting aside, many Americans are at risk for too little manganese, rather than too much. It is estimated that 37 percent of Americans have low-manganese intake.

Mad Cow Disease: Is It a Concern?

Mad cow disease is the commonly used name for bovine spongiform encephalopathy (BSE), a serious disease affecting cows. BSE is a degenerative neurologic disorder that most recently emerged in Europe in the 1980s. Its appearance in cows has been traced back to the use of diseased sheep parts in cattle feed, since sheep can suffer from a similar disease. But until BSE began appearing in cows, farmers did not know the disease could pass between these two species.

What does a cow's disease mean to you? Well, it seems this disease can also transfer between the species of cow and human. The BSE-related form of this disease that strikes humans is called variant Creutzfeldt-Jakob disease (vCJD), and several cases have been found in Europe.

Chondroitin is manufactured from bovine (cow) trachea. Theoretically, BSE could be transmitted through cow-derived products, such as chondroitin supplements. However, there are numerous safeguards in place to ensure the safety of beef products. For starters, the Food and Drug Administration (FDA) has import restrictions prohibiting the importation of beef or other cow parts for use in foods or dietary supplements from countries with known cases of BSE. Furthermore, protective steps are taken in the manufacturing process, including the use of cows only from certified non-BSE countries and the enzymatic digestion of all proteins (the infective part causing BSE is a protein fragment).

So the bottom line is that you should be no more concerned about the risk of vCJD from dietary supplements than you are from the meat you might eat. Meat and supplements derived from animal sources are held to the same standards to protect the public from vCJD.

Shellfish Allergies: Proceed with Caution

If you have an allergy to shellfish, you should avoid glucosamine supplements. Many glucosamine products are manufactured from crab shells, and there is a slight risk that some of the crabmeat could in-advertently be included along with the shell during the manufacturing process. Even though the risk is small, erring on the side of safety means avoiding these supplements.

Always a Good Idea to Consult Your Doctor

You don't need a doctor's prescription to buy the dietary supplements glucosamine and chondroitin, or the others discussed in this book, such as vitamin C, vitamin D, and SAMe. However, it is a good idea to consult with your physician before treating your osteoarthritis.

For example, it's important to ensure that osteoarthritis is the source of your joint symptoms, rather than a different joint condition such as bursitis, gout, lupus, or rheumatoid arthritis. The chart on the following page shows the main symptoms of these different disorders.

CONDITION	MAIN SYMPTOMS
Bursitis	Pain and swelling in a joint caused by inflammation of a bursa, a saclike membrane between bone and tissues near a joint. Often traced to a sports injury.
Gout	Metabolic disorder most frequently affecting the big toe. Sudden, sharp, painful attack of tenderness in the joint. Most common in men over age forty who have a family history of this condition.
Lupus	Joint pain, redness, and swelling, that varies from day to day, most often affecting the fingers and wrists. Chest pain, coughing, fatigue, rashes, and sunlight sensitivity often present. Women in their twenties and thirties are most often affected.
Osteoarthritis	Joint pain, limited range of motion, stiffness. Usually starts in just one joint, often after an injury or overuse. More common with increasing age.
Rheumatoid arthritis	Autoimmune disorder, with joint inflammation as key manifestation. Loss of motion, pain, redness comes and goes.

CONCLUSION

If dietary supplements have a good chance of helping you and cause no harm—why wouldn't you give them a try? Such is the case with glucosamine and chondroitin for osteoarthritis. The argument for trying these supplements is bolstered by the fact that they can replace, or at least reduce, your use of NSAID medications that have a clearly documented potential for harm.

Sir William Osler, a nineteenth century British physician, stated his disappointment over not having a viable treatment for arthritis: "When a patient with arthritis walks in the front door, I feel like leaving out the back door." In the many years since he made that statement, not much has changed in terms of any success for conventional medicine in treating arthritis. This lack of success is not for lack of trying. Most of those with arthritis are overwhelmed by one side-effect-provoking medication after another. But until one of these drugs is able to treat arthritis without excessive side effects, arthritis will remain conventional medicine's failure.

This is where glucosamine, chondroitin, and other dietary supplements come in. While these supplements can't promise to be a magic bullet, they do have a lot to offer—from decreasing reliance on NSAIDs to doing what doctors can't: relieving the inflammation, mobility impairments, and pain of arthritis while actually promoting the growth of new, healthy cartilage.

If you are among the more than one in ten Americans currently suffering from osteoarthritis, relief cannot come to soon. Give glucosamine and/or chondroitin a try.

SELECTED
REFERENCES

Bourgeois, P, Chales, G, Dehais, J, et al. Efficacy and tolerability of chondroitin sulfate 1200 mg/day vs chondroitin sulfate 3 x 400 mg/day vs placebo. *Osteoarthritis and Cartilage*, 1998; 6SupplA:25–30.

Conrozier, T. Anti-arthrosis treatments: efficacy and tolerance of chondroitin sulfates (CS 4&6). *Presse Medicale*, 1998; 27:1862–1865.

Das, A, Hammad, TA. Efficacy of a combination of FCHG49® glucosamine hydrochloride, TRH122® low molecular weight sodium chondroitin sulfate and manganese ascorbate in the management of knee osteoarthritis. *Osteoarthritis and Cartilage*, 2000; 8:343–350.

Deal, CL, Moskowitz, RW. Nutraceuticals as therapeutic agents in osteoarthritis. *Rheumatic Diseases Clinics of North America*, 1999; 25:379–395.

Ezzo, J, Hadhazy, V, Birch, S, et al. Acupuncture for osteoarthritis of the knee: a systematic review. *Arthritis and Rheumatism*, 2001; 44:819–825.

Flynn, MA. The effect of folate and cobalamin on osteoarthritic hands. *Journal of the American College of Nutrition*, August 1994; 13:351–356.

Gaby, AR. Natural treatments for osteoarthritis. *Alternative Medicine Review*, 1999; 4:330–341.

Hoffer, LJ, Kaplan, LN, Hamadeh, MJ, et al. Sulfate could mediate the therapeutic effect of glucosamine sulfate. *Metabolism*, 2001; 50:767–770.

Jonas, WB, Rapoza, CP, Blair, WF. The effect of niacinamide on osteoarthritis: a pilot study. *Inflammation Research*, 1996; 45:330–344.

Kaufman, W. The use of vitamin therapy to reverse certain concomitants of aging. *Journal of the American Geriatric Society,* 1955; 3:927–936.

Leffler, CT, Philippi, AF, Leffler, SG, et al. Glucosamine, chondroitin, and manganese ascorbate for degenerative joint disease of the knee or low back: a randomized, double-blind, placebo-controlled pilot study. *Military Medicine,* 1999; 164:85–91.

Lippiello, L, Woodward, J, Karpman, R, et al. In vivo chondroprotection and metabolic synergy of glucosamine and chondroitin sulfate. *Clinical Orthopaedics and Related Research,* 2000; 381:229–240.

McAlindon, TE, LaValley, MP, Gulin, JP, et al. Glucosamine and chondroitin for treatment of osteoarthritis. *Journal of the American Medical Association,* 2000; 283:1469–1475.

McAlindon, TE, Jacques, P, Zhang, Y, et al. Do antioxidant micronutrients protect against the development and progression of knee osteoarthritis? *Arthritis & Rheumatism,* 1996; 39:648–656.

Reginster, JY, Deroisy, R, Rovati, L, et al. Long-term effects of glucosamine sulphate on osteoarthritis progression: a randomized, placebo-controlled clinical trial. *Lancet,* 2001; 357:251–256.

Russell, AL. Glycoaminoglycan (GAG) deficiency in protective barrier as an underlying, primary cause of ulcer-ative colitis, Crohn's disease, interstitial cystitis, and pos-sibly Reiter's syndrome. *Medical Hypotheses,* 1999; 52: 297–301.

Tapadinhas, MJ, Rivera, IC, Binamini, AA. Oral glucosamine sulfate in the management of arthrosis: report on a multi-centre open investigation in Portugal. *Pharmatherapeutica,* 1982; 3:157–168.

Thie, NM, Prasad, NG, Major, PW. Evaluation of glucos-amine sulfate compared to ibuprofen for the treatment of temporomandibular joint osteoarthritis: a randomized double-blind, placebo-controlled 3 month clinical trial. *Journal of Rheumatology,* 2001; 28: 1347–1355.

Towheed, TE, Anastassiades, TP, Shea, B, et al. Glucosamine therapy for treating osteoarthritis (Cochrane Review). *Cochrane Database of Systematic Reviews,* 2001; 1:CD002946.

Other Books and Resources

Lininger, SL. (Editor-in-chief). *The Natural Pharmacy.* Prima Health, Rocklin, CA, 1999.

Somer, E. *Age-Proof Your Body.* William Morrow and Company, New York, 1998.

GreatLife Magazine
Consumer magazine with articles on vitamins, minerals, herbs, and foods.
Available for free at many health and natural food stores.

Let's Live Magazine
Consumer magazine with emphasis on the health benefits of vitamins, minerals, and herbs.
Customer service:
1-800-676-4333
P.O. Box 74908
Los Angeles, CA 90004
Subscriptions: 12 issues per year, $19.95 in the U.S.; $31.95 outside the U.S.

Physical Magazine
Magazine oriented to body builders and other serious athletes.
Customer service:
1-800-676-4333
P.O. Box 74908
Los Angeles, CA 90004
Subscriptions: 12 issues per year, $19.95 in the U.S.; $31.95 outside the U.S.

The Nutrition Reporter™ newsletter

Monthly newsletter that summarizes recent medical research on vitamins, minerals, and herbs.

Customer service:

P.O. Box 30246

Tucson, AZ 85751-0246

e-mail: jack@thenutritionreporter.com

www.nutritionreporter.com

Subscriptions: $26 per year (12 issues) in the U.S.; $32 U.S. or $48 CNC for Canada; $38 for other countries

Arthritis Foundation

P.O. Box 7669

Atlanta, Georgia 30357-0669

1-800-283-7800

www.arthritis.org

National Institute of Arthritis and Musculo-skeletal and Skin Diseases

Information Clearinghouse

National Institutes of Health

1 AMS Circle

Bethesda, Maryland 20892-3675

1-877-22-NIAMS (toll-free)

e-mail: niamsinfo@mail.nih.gov

www.nih.gov/niams

INDEX

Printed in the USA
CPSIA information can be obtained
at www.ICGtesting.com
JSHW011257021023
49511JS00004B/94